The Language of Illness

First published in 2020 by
Liberties Press
1 Terenure Place | Terenure | Dublin 6W | Ireland
www.libertiespress.com

Distributed in the United States and Canada by
Casemate IPM | 1950 Lawrence Rd | Havertown | Pennsylvania 19083 | USA
Tel: 001 610 853 9131
www.casemateipm.com

2 4 6 8 10 9 7 5 3 1
A CIP record for this title is available from the British Library.
Cover image reproduced courtesy of Project Twins: Oh Great!, acrylic on paper, site-specific installation, '2012 Living/Loss: The Experience of Illness in Art' at The Lewis
Glucksman Gallery, University College Cork, 2012-13

The Language of
Illness

Fergus Shanahan

for Nora

Contents

Preface   vii

1.   Introduction: When Crisis Meets Routine   1

2.   Disease-speak and Its Distancing Effect   10

    Replacing Familiar with Unfamiliar – Medicine's Misnomers – Crotchets – Clichés – Reforming the Medical Record – The Bad Historian – Slang and Codes – Abbreviations – Name My Condition – The Literary Alternative

3.   The Illness Words   26

    Hope – Suffering – Loss – Fear – Anger – Denial – Degradation and Shame – Loneliness and Aloneness – Disbelief and Dismissal – Gain – Trust – Humour

4.   Waiting, Uncertainty and Time   54

5.   It's the Way You Say It   64

    Epiphanies – Chitchat – Loose Talk – Questions – Real-speak – Framing the Question – Framing Risk – Leading Questions – Interruptions – Mending Mindsets – Coaching Not Coaxing – Plain Language and Clean Language – No Claptrap – Social Media Medicine

6.   No Words, Just Silent Signals   83

    The Body Doesn't Lie – Small Behaviours – Looking the Part – Digital Doc and the Third Presence – The Most Underrated Clinical Discipline – The Importance of Silences – Doctoring as a Performance Art – Style – Touching – Presence – An Important Resource

7.   Healing Words, Hurting Words   101

    The Barracuda at the Front Office – Dr Nocebo and Dr Placebo – Metaphoric Medic – Who's Afraid of Susan Sontag? – The Personal Metaphor – Dappled Things – Sticks and Stones . . . and Stigma – Stigma Stories from Sick Doctors – Science and Stigma – Tell It Slant

8. Language Gaps and Words that Get in the Way   119

The All-clear – Hyper or Tense, or Both? – The 'Difficult' Patient – Pain Scales – Softer or Stronger Words – 'Second' or 'Secondary' Victims – The Tyranny of a Positive Attitude – End-of-life Language

9. Words that Turn People into Patients   129

The Dangers of Labels – What's Normal? – Medical Chic – The Medicine-seeking Animal – Maverick Priest – Non-diseases – Medically Unexplained Symptoms – The Most Neglected Word in Healthcare – Clever Words Create Vulnerable Patients – From Mislabels to Mistreatment – Different Words Change the Treatment – Wellness Language

10. The Weight of a Word: Caring, Dignity and Empathy   145

11. Language, Logic, Policy and Poor Public Health Messages   155

If You Have Symptoms, It's Diagnosis Not Screening – Is Everything a Risk Factor for Something? – Misleading Misnomer – Obesity Distorted by Bad Language – Antibiotic Resistance – Changing the Narrative on Vaccination – Weary from Awareness

12. The Patient and the System   165

Politico-speak – Forbidden Words – Preferred Words – Words of Deflection – Gobbledegook – Patient v. System – The Sophisticated Deception

13. The Language of Plagues and Pandemics   176

Pandemic Parlance – Finding the Personal Stories – Misnomers and Metaphors – Binary Language and Logic – A Communications Emergency – A Pandemic Pause To Consider Our Place in Nature

Epilogue   186
Notes   187
Bibliography   197
Acknowledgements   214
Index   216

Preface

This is the book I would like to have read when I set out on a life of doctoring. It is also the kind of book that might have helped me as a parent desperately seeking to help a seriously sick young man. This book is *about* patients and carers, and it is *for* patients and carers. It is about how words shape the thoughts, decisions and judgements doctors make on behalf of their patients. It is also about the inadequacy of language to express what it feels like to be ill, and the distancing effect that language may have on the patient-doctor interaction. Patients frequently feel they speak a language different from that of their doctor. This is unnecessary. One of the great paradoxes of modern medicine is that most advances have shortened the time patients and doctors spend together; mismatched language needlessly diminishes the effective use of that time.

Conversations between patients and doctors are the basis of effective healthcare but doctors use disease-words whereas patients speak illness-language. Illness is what it feels like to have a disease. It is the lived experience of disease. I've learned to accept that technical language is occasionally required when communicating complex ideas, but I'm suspicious of words that require explanation, particularly words that can easily be replaced with ordinary words.

Ultracrepidarian. That's the title of the picture in my mind, the work of a whimsical Irish graphic art duo, the Project Twins, who generate images to represent the meanings of curious words. *Ultracrepidarian* sounds like it might be a word to mock the ageing mind and body. It isn't, but it is a reminder of the importance of honesty and humility in medicine. The word means: giving opinions and advice on matters outside of one's knowledge. I get lots of humbling reminders from my children and my patients. I also have my ego punctured regularly by the peer-review process in medical science. My credentials for this book are that I have played several roles in different illness stories. I've studied disease and experienced illness. I'm expert enough to be wary of experts.

Effective communication and dialogue does not come easily to most people. It requires practice and self-reflection. Careful consideration of the words we use, not only in clinical encounters but in all avenues of medicine, is probably the most important lesson in professional life. In an era when the scale and pace of medical science exceeds the capacity of the human mind, doctors face new challenges to their decision-making and thinking. An avalanche of technology, including big data, machine-learning, algorithms, decision-trees and guidelines, with an expectation to practise evidence-based everything, threatens to change forever the way doctors interact with patients. While medical schools rightly struggle to improve the effectiveness of doctor-patient communication, the poverty and inadequacy of the language of medicine has changed little.

Words do more than help patients and doctors communicate. Words can inspire, inform and transform; they can be therapeutic; and they are a reflection on the art, science and business of doctoring. Words may also do harm. To borrow from George Orwell: the slovenliness of our language 'makes it easier for us to have foolish thoughts'. Why then do so many doctors, health service managers and policymakers take words for granted?

This is not a manual for patients to interpret doctor-speak: there are plenty of those around. Nor is it a book about communication skills for doctors, although it is not unrelated to that. Rather, it is a plea for more critical appraisal of illness-language. It looks at language and logic that can help or hinder patients, and calls for more effective use of conversation-time between patients and doctors. The book is intended for two audiences, each of which approaches illness from a different perspective: doctors, nurses and other healthcare professionals, on the one hand, and patients' relatives, friends and loved ones, on the other. These differ in expertise as well as perspective, but need not be separated by language.

Who should read this book? It's for anyone who cares about caring.

1

ക്കി

Introduction: When Crisis Meets Routine

What do you say to someone who becomes seriously ill? What words? How to behave? Why is it awkward?

One of the peculiarities of illness is how unprepared most of us are when it strikes – despite the certainty that, sooner or later, everyone becomes part of an illness story. For all its universality, illness is one of the few truly unique events in a life. Illness is the lived experience of disease. It is deeply personal, and no two individuals with the same disease will experience illness in the same way. Unlike in earlier times, illness is now more likely to be long-lived and chronic. This is due to medical advances, and an increase in the prevalence of chronic disorders linked with lifestyles in socio-economically developed countries.

Most illness-stories still begin as a crisis, with few people having any advance warning about what it feels like to be sick or disabled. Since thinking comes before judgements, decisions and actions, the language that shapes our thinking about illness needs precision and accuracy. Moreover, if storytelling is part of healing and coping, then most people are disadvantaged, unfamiliar with the words which are needed. Nor do they have the language to help others cope with illness. This creates awkwardness, and contributes to the isolation and suffering which is experienced with many illnesses.

Part of the problem is the disease-focused nature of medical language used by doctors, healthcare systems and the media, which avoids illness words like *suffering, stigma, fear* and *anger*. Why is it that so many patients are fearful of telling their doctors the whole story? Many feel assaulted by harsh new words: it seems to them to be an attack on their vocabulary and a challenge to their sense of self. The distancing effect of medical language and jargon is discussed in Chapter 2. Throughout this book, the word *disease* refers to the objective evidence that something is wrong, whereas *illness* is what the patient with the disease experiences.

Modern medicine has become expert at rescuing patients from acute, life-threatening diseases. Doctors can also control most chronic diseases, including many cancers, but helping patients to deal with the illness-experience of those diseases, is orders of magnitude more challenging. 'It's hard, perhaps impossibly hard, to be a good doctor', wrote former editor of the *British Medical Journal* Dr Richard Smith in 2012. Finding a good doctor, according to Smith, is 'like finding a good lover: there are lots of anecdotes but no data'. Smith was intrigued by an essay entitled 'The Patient Examines the Doctor', which was written by the literary critic Anatole Broyard while he was dying from prostate cancer and which appears in Broyard's book *Intoxicated by My Illness*. Broyard wanted more than technical competence from his doctor – 'I want my doctor to have magic as well as medical ability' – and humorously listed desirable attributes for the ideal doctor, to which no single doctor of unlimited talent could aspire. 'To get to my body, my doctor has to get to my character. He has to go through my soul.' *Soul* is a word which is seldom heard in doctor-speak, and doesn't feature today in medical literature, except when institutional care is described as soulless. Institutions have no soul, but people do. For anthropologist and psychiatrist Arthur Kleinman, this old-world word, rich with religious connotation, represents the 'innermost existential centre to our being'. Kleinman believes that 'we need soul to specify the human quality at the heart of care in order to animate the souls of patients, family members and clinicians'.

Another description of what it takes to be a good doctor was captured by Dr Robert Brook in an article in the *Journal of the American Medical Association* in 2010, entitled: 'A physician = science + emotion + passion'.

Doctors need science to think about *disease*, and they need emotion and passion to address the *illness* experienced by people with the disease. From emotion and passion, come compassion, kindness and humanity. One more item may be added to that formula: Physician = science + emotion + passion and . . . curiosity.

When crisis meets routine, routine needs to be curious. Curiosity keeps medical minds fresh, engaged and motivated to try to understand illness as well as disease. Caring *for* patients means caring *about* patients, and that is driven by curiosity.

The context in which a patient consults a doctor is fraught with multiple asymmetries. From the outset, the relationship is imbalanced. The stakes are higher for the patient than for the doctor. The patient is boss, but seldom feels that way. The patient's main level of control is in the selection of the doctor – although this has been lost in some healthcare systems, such as Britain's NHS. The doctor is servant but, otherwise, is in a controlling position. Doctors don't see patients at their best. However, the greatest barrier to an effective patient-doctor relationship is a disparity in language.

Patient	Doctor
Crisis	Routine
Illness-focused	Disease-focused
Subjective	Objective
Strange surroundings	Usual environment
Extraordinary event	Ordinary occurrence
Plays the sick role	A performance art
Unsure, loss of confidence	Composed, confident
Unprepared, nervous	Ready and trained
Threatened sense of self-identity	Self-assured
Lacks information, sense of helplessness	Possesses knowledge, experience
Bears some responsibility for self-care	Has greater share of responsibility for outcome
Disrobed, disfigured or hospital-gown humiliated	Uniform, elegant
Seeks wisdom	Commands the words, expertise and jargon
Judgement impaired by sickness	Judgement unbiased
Altered perception of time	Time-conscious, rushed
Chooses the doctor, where possible	Does not select patients
Master	Servant

The Asymmetries of the Doctor-patient Relationship

Patients frequently feel that they speak a language which is different from that of their doctors. Too often, little attention is given to the illness-words with which patients are concerned. The illness-words are discussed in Chapter 3. Some words, like *loss, fear* and *shame,* relate to aspects of illness which are often poorly dealt with, or ignored, by modern medicine. My thoughts on these words have been mined from conversations I have had over the years with patients, and from a variety of illness-memoirs. The illness-memoir has become established as a distinct genre in modern literature and the subject of several scholarly critiques. Those by Kathlyn Conway, Thomas Couser, Arthur Frank and Anne Hunsaker Hawkins, I found especially informative. Illness-memoirs naturally vary in quality, but each represents a story that is unique in the true sense of that word. Many illness-memoirs are stories of triumph over adversity, whereas others tell a story of loss and disruption. Some authors have found that the chaotic, non-linear or overlapping nature of the experience of illness cannot be captured adequately in the writing process. For these reasons, I have taken a complementary approach by extracting key illness-words and deliberating on them.

No doubt some illnesses are likely to be particularly linked with certain feelings, such as a sense of shame, denial or despair, but other words are common to almost all illness-stories. These include waiting, uncertainty and time – which are examined in Chapter 4. For example, the perception of time changes for those who are ill. The past evokes sadness and regret, the future is uncertain, and the present seems to slow down, even as it continues apace for doctors and other carers.

Of course, dialogue between patient and doctor is not a normal social situation. It is more akin to a duet, in which the patient leads, setting the tune and tempo, for the doctor to respond to and improvise around. When the doctor's improvisations are effective, there is jazz, even harmony. Occasionally, the patient and doctor fall out of tune, and there is noise. Language, both verbal and non-verbal, can reduce the distance between doctor and patient or, if misused, can amplify the difficulties. While doctors need to pay more attention to the words they use and how they use them (Chapter 5), the non-verbal exchanges with their patients are often more important. Sick people are unconsciously hyper-sensitive to non-verbal cues that signal the concern and interest (or lack thereof) of others: the touch of a caring hand or the comfort of a reassuring smile (discussed in Chapter 6).

Doctors usually know what's wrong with a patient within the first minutes of their conversation. But the exchange accomplishes more than assembling facts: when handled properly, doctor-patient dialogue may be therapeutic. Sadly, it is often a lost opportunity to promote healing, and may even increase suffering. The healing and hurting words of medicine are discussed in Chapter 7, and the inadequacy of words, and language gaps in health and medicine, are addressed in Chapter 8.

The language of medicine is full of paradox and ambiguity. The greatest paradox of modern medicine – doing better, feeling worse – was famously identified by Roy Porter in the opening lines of his medical history of humanity: 'These are strange times, when we are healthier than ever but more anxious about our health.' Misuse of language has contributed to the transition from health-consciousness to health-anxiety, with the creation of new disorders for commercial gain, and the over-medicalisation of society. Words that turn people into patients are discussed in Chapter 9.

Another paradox highlighted by Professor Arthur Kleinman is that medicine invests little in caregiving, yet it is central to what it means to be human and is 'core to health professionals' motivations and identity'. Since contemporary fiction represents a faithful historic record, it seems reasonable to consider how the performance of doctors has been assessed by the great storytellers. Judging doctors is a bit like assessing curates and their eggs: you get some good ones and some bad ones, each being good in parts. Doctors probably reflect the society from which they are drawn. Moreover, fictional doctors reflect the context of their times. However, those who have fared well are outnumbered by those portrayed in a poor light, exhibiting coldness instead of compassion. *Empathy* is the more popular word today for what patients want from their doctors and other caregivers. The word is relatively new in medical and related literature.

I am always suspicious of a word that requires explanation. True empathy is unusual, usually unrealistic, and occasionally undesirable. I will argue that the word is an unnecessary substitute for the more attainable and realistic attributes of kindness and compassion. Doctors cannot know exactly how you feel, or what it feels like to be sick. 'It is a pity that getting all the diseases cannot be made part of the medical training,' lamented Dr David Mendel in his book *Proper Doctoring*. True empathy is vanishingly rare, in part because illness is experienced differently by different patients, and in part because it is impossible to know what it feels like to be ill if one has not had the same experience. This was acknowledged centuries ago by the poet John Donne, who wrote from a patient's perspective:

> Diseases which we never felt in ourselves come but to a compassion of others that have endured them; nay, compassion itself comes to no great degree if we have not felt in some proportion in ourselves that which we lament and condole in another.

Caring, dignity and *empathy* are words loaded with paradox and ambiguity, and are examined in detail in Chapter 10.

Of course, illness-stories are played out beyond the confines of hospitals and doctors' offices. Everyone has a role in the story of an illness, but the way we play that role can mitigate or accentuate the ordeal of illness. How to behave with the ill? 'This is hard I know,' conceded the poet Julia Darling, who died from breast cancer:

> try not to ignore the ill, or to scurry
> past, muttering about a bus, the bank
> — 'How to behave with the ill', Julia Darling (1956-2005)

This process begins with confronting our own awkwardness and a determination not to indulge in self-serving contrivances that permit us to stay away. It is difficult to find something to say that does not offend sick people, to find words that are kind, or at least not unkind; but words are not essential. 'I don't know what to say' is the honest thing to say. On the awkwardness of encounters with strangers or friends, and the social isolation of illness, philosopher Havi Carel, who has a serious lung disease, commented: 'what I have learned from my illness is that in times of hardship, grief, and loss, there is no need for original illuminating phrases. There is nothing to say other than the most banal stuff.'

Suffering is inescapable, but some aspects of illness are avoidable products of the behaviour of others and the attitudes of society to illness. Although the experience of illness is never the same in different people with the same disease, there is remarkable consensus from the stories of those with serious illness on what to do, or not do, when meeting a person or family dealing with illness. Most important: try not to ignore the ill. The rationalisation that nothing can be done is no refuge, nor is the convenient assumption that the sick wish to be alone. Engage. Be there. Don't assume that the sick wish to avoid the difficult subject or to be distracted with idle chatter: sometimes their illness is the *only* thing they wish to talk about. If invited, don't be afraid to touch; everyone needs a hug sometimes.

The sick and the disabled are sensitive to subtle changes in the behaviour of others in response to their misfortune. Words and gestures adopt uncommon significance. Compassion is always appreciated and can be sensed, but the sick do not need silences to be filled with words. Companionship, or simply being there, is sufficient support. Don't parrot any clichés or sentimentality. Humour may seem utterly misplaced, but sick people often report comic episodes, particularly with old friends. For example, during rehabilitation in hospital after his stroke, the poet Seamus Heaney was visited by his friend, the playwright Brian Friel, who had also suffered a stroke a year earlier. Friel remarked to Heaney: 'different strokes for different folks'.

Christopher Hitchens found that 'the presence of friends' was his chief consolation after he was diagnosed with oesophageal cancer, but considered whether there should be 'ground rules' on etiquette for how sympathisers and sufferers of cancer should interact. His proposed etiquette handbook would provide guidelines to address the 'inevitable awkwardness in diplomatic relations between Tumourtown and its neighbours'. He was assailed with advice and rumours of cures which were well intended but tedious. Referring to the lingua franca of Tumourville as 'dull and difficult', he found jaded clichés and exhortations intended to boost morale 'vaguely depressing'. Likewise, he declares that grave illness makes one suspicious of popular expressions of received wisdom regarding health. He recommends that we avoid them. In much the same way that one could die of encouragement in Tinseltown, Hitchens thought that in Tumourtown one could expire from sheer *advice*. Vacuous stories of others with the same, or similar, illnesses do not provide much succour to distressed patients trying to cope with a grave illness. Anatole Broyard also wrote of being regaled with the stories of others after his diagnosis with metastatic prostate cancer: 'Storytelling seems to be a natural reaction to illness. People bleed stories, and I've become a bloodbank of them.' Storytelling is for the one who is ill, not for the visitor.

Kate Bowler, a young woman with late-stage colon cancer, also listed the *storytellers* among her short list of what should be avoided when speaking with anyone with a serious illness. Worse than the storytellers, are the *minimisers*. Never say 'It could have been worse' or 'Well, at least you don't have . . . '. Similarly, don't be a philosopher – the sick don't need greeting-card-type clichés ('God needs an angel') – and never try to explain the meaning of illness ('Everything happens for a reason' or 'God works in mysterious ways'). Be careful with language and war metaphors ('your battle with illness'), because it is not within the control of the sufferer. As Christopher Hitchens protested, he wasn't in a battle with his own cancer: 'I'm not fighting or battling cancer – it's fighting me.'

It is sufficient to show that you care by being with the person who is ill. Sustained engagement, even when nothing practical can be done, is to bear witness with moral solidarity. Its importance becomes evident when it is absent. *Presence* is how Dr Arthur Kleinman succinctly describes this core component of caring. The importance of presence was captured by Seamus Heaney in his poem 'Miracle', written while he was recovering from the stroke mentioned above. In a gesture of gratitude to those in the background – 'the ones who have known him all along' – Heaney acknowledged the ordinary people who support by their presence: 'be mindful of them as they stand and wait'. 'Human presence is the important part of visiting,' wrote Lucy Grealy, whose mother would quickly dispense with news and information about Lucy's health and then spend the entire visit knitting. This was the 'Visitor Extraordinaire' for Lucy: 'her body occupied a space close to my body, but it didn't ask anything of it'. Other visitors, in contrast – including her father – were uneasy, awkward and uncomfortable with silences, 'when all I wanted was for them to sit down, relax, not say a word'.

Language-gaps are not limited to the sick and their carers: poor use of language spills into public health policy. (Mixed, confused and mistaken public health messages are discussed in Chapter 11.) Misunderstandings abound. An example is the failure of health authorities and the media to explain the distinction between screening for disease in people with no symptoms, and diagnosis of disease in patients with symptoms. This has misled, alarmed, and undermined public confidence in many screening programs. Flawed language also contributes to ineffectual campaigns addressing obesity, antibiotic resistance and vaccination uptake. In some instances, public health ventures have reinforced rather than reduced the stigmatising effect of illness.

The patient-doctor relationship remains the keystone of healthcare, but this relationship is continually changing. Patients need time and wisdom from their doctors, but are no longer dependent on doctors for information. For chronic disease, the consultation will become a collaboration, and the doctor's role will become more akin to that of a coach helping the patient navigate the system of healthcare. Words that sell the system, protect and perpetuate the status quo, obfuscate, and occasionally deceive, are discussed in Chapter 12.

The real heroes of healthcare are on the frontline. In the background are the hidden weaknesses and inequities of the system. These are revealed in times of major societal threat, such as that posed by a pandemic. Since a pandemic is a communications emergency as well as a health and economic crises, the language of pandemics is discussed in Chapter 13.

2

❧❧❧

Disease-speak and Its Distancing Effect

'Words, words, words, I'm so sick of words.'

— Eliza Doolittle[1]

Replacing the Familiar with the Unfamiliar – Medicine's Misnomers – Crotchets – Clichés – Reforming the Medical Record – Bad Historian – Slang and Codes – Abbreviations – Name My Condition – The Literary Alternative

Ten thousand! That's the number of words a student learns in the first year of training to be a doctor. The number may eventually exceed fifty thousand. Becoming a physician is like learning a second language, except that the average vocabulary acquired by students of modern languages seldom reaches five thousand.[2] Great battalions of big words, worn like armour, embolden a doctor's image and enhance the mystique of medicine. Most of these words need to be challenged. Even the first principle of medicine burned onto the consciousness of all medical trainees – *first do no harm* – is usually written in the Latin, *primum non nocere*. Most medical students have a vague idea that the expression was first uttered by Hippocrates, but he was Greek, didn't write in Latin, and nowhere does the term appear in the Hippocratic oath.[3] Once, Latin was the language of medicine (*lingua medica*); this was a time when medicine was ineffective and limited to the prescription of potions, purges and placebos, and a doctor's skill was one of eloquent performance. A different kind of cleverness with words is now required. Many traditional medical words are effete and unnecessary, and have long outlived their usefulness. Some are obstacles to effective communication with the modern patient.

It takes a brave and perceptive patient to question the shallowness of medical words. Molly Bloom has this to say about her gynaecologist in her famous soliloquy imagined by James Joyce in *Ulysses*:

where do those old fellows get all the words they have . . . I wouldn't trust him too far.

Mathew Arnold rejects conventional deathbed wisdom in his poem 'A Wish', and dismisses the doctor from the sickroom:

> Nor bring, to see cease to live,
> Some doctor full of phrase and fame,
> To shake his sapient head and give
> The Ill he cannot cure a name.

Similarly, in Margaret Edson's play *W;t, the* misfortunate Professor Vivian Bearing, who is undergoing chemotherapy for advanced ovarian cancer, tells the audience:

> I want to know what the doctors mean when they . . . anatomise me. . . . They possess a more potent arsenal of terminology than I. My only defence is the acquisition of vocabulary.

The foreign vocabulary of medicine is at the heart of Lorrie Moore's story of a mother's struggle to cope with her little boy's illness with cancer. *All the words are like blows*, she thinks. She says all the words aloud to herself: *sarcoma, metastases, Hickman catheter, lesions.* The mother, a writer and teacher, is desperate to regain control, and needs to master the words. 'Is that apostrophe "s" or "s" apostrophe?' she asks, when the doctor says her child has Wilms' tumour, 'as if it were the most normal thing in the world'. He is also unsure about the spelling.

Julia Darling, who died of breast cancer, mocked medical words in witty prose and poetry. In a playful poem written to her doctor 'to complain about these words you have given me . . . they tick like bombs and overpower my sweet-tasting words', she juxtaposes the doctor's ugly words (*lymphatic, nodal, progressive, metastatic)* with the ordinary ones she uses herself (*orange, bus, coffee, June, lollipop, monkey, lip*).

There are, of course, occasional pleasant-sounding words in medicine. I like, for example, words describing sounds, such as *borborygmi* (abdominal gurgling), *murmur, bruit* (sounds in the heart or blood vessels) and *whispering pectoriloquy* (enhanced voice sound heard with stethoscope over an area of lung consolidation from pneumonia). I also like pronouncing *intussusception* (telescoping of the bowel) and *bezoar* (foreign-body vegetable matter in the stomach), and find the terms for some nutritional deficiencies musically appealing, such as *beri beri* and *kwashiorkor*. I dislike *marasmus,* however. *Tsutsugamushi* is delightfully exotic, but it isn't a Japanese gourmet dish; rather, it is an insect-borne bacterial infection of humans! From non-medical English, but often applicable in medicine, I like the word *insouciant*. Delightful-sounding as these words may be, they are unnecessary.

The expansion of vocabulary which accompanies illness has fascinated many authors. During treatment for leukaemia, the essayist Sinéad Gleeson mused on the symbolism of blood, and on the banalities of repeated blood-tests. *Vacuettes*, the brand name for the colour-coded vacuum-primed tubes into which her blood was aspirated, was a useful distraction from needlesticks: 'The Vacuettes – great name for an all-girl punk band,' she said to herself, 'or vacuette could be the name of a French heroine in a romance novel or slang for dim mean-girls.' Similarly, Allessandra Colaianni found humour in medical jargon. imagining pop musicians and rock bands with medical names such as *The Notochords*, *The Haemophiliacs* (punks) and *The Obturators* (heavy metal). In a bittersweet account of her time as a medical student, the language of medicine actually became a 'bridge to the world outside medical school'. She defected to this 'parallel universe' to pursue a career in theatre. While acknowledging the need to use certain words in order to be specific in medical language, Colaianni noted that other terms seemed to make things more obscure rather than clearer.

REPLACING THE FAMILIAR WITH THE UNFAMILIAR

The first thing that happens when students go to medical school is that they are quickly taught how to replace the familiar with the unfamiliar. This begins the process of creating distance between the ordinary world of their future patients and their new, medical world. Some technical jargon is, of course, necessary, and a mastery of the names for a multitude of obscure anatomic details facilitates communication among doctors, but much of the medical vocabulary is unnecessary. Is it useful or necessary to refer to an itch as *pruritus* (usually misspelled as a *pruritis*)? Why bother to refer to a nosebleed as *epistaxis*, jaundice as *icterus*, and a runny nose as *rhinorrhoea*? On the other hand, *nasal catarrh* is preferable to *snot*. Likewise, potential embarrassment can be overcome by occasional medicalisation of words, such as *stools* or *faeces* in preference to a shorter word for the same thing. But surely, *haemorrhage* adds nothing useful over the simpler word, bleeding. This humble word has been further transformed by gynaecologists and obstetricians for menstrual bleeding (*menorrhagia*), and for some unfortunate women more terrifying categories of menstrual bleeding have been devised (*metrorrhagia* and *menometrorrhagia*). These words are not needed and do not deserve an explanation.[4]

Every speciality within medicine has enthusiastically contributed marvellous examples of obscure and unnecessary words to rename the familiar and the ordinary. The skin-doctors (dermatologists) surely take the prize for the most flamboyant use of Latin descriptors for rashes. These marvellous words impress and bewilder patients. Almost everything has a fancy name. Even the most ordinary of findings, such as skin discoloration from the heat of an open fire or a hot-water bottle, is given a Latin descriptor (*erythema ab igne*). This is harmless, but other terms are often misleading, even frightening. For example, *pyoderma gangrenosum* is a completely inaccurate descriptor for what is actually a serious, disfiguring immune-mediated disorder that requires specialist precision therapeutics.

The precise meaning of medical words and phrases was a subject that concerned Richard Asher, one of the great thinkers of twentieth-century medicine. Asher pointed out that medical words may confuse as well as clarify the subject they purport to describe. Words may inflate the apparent importance of illnesses of dubious clinical significance; they may perpetuate non-existent disorders or fail to identify adequately others that do exist. We will see later, in Chapter 9, how words may be exploited to medicalise non-existent disorders for commercial purposes. Unfortunately, medical words are difficult to change. To borrow from Thomas Payne, 'a long habit of not thinking a thing wrong, gives it a superficial appearance of being right'. Asher's analysis showed that the words used in clinical medicine continue to distort textbook descriptions and clinical thinking.

Curiously, while doctors acquire the vocabulary of diseases, they seem to abandon the illness words. Scan any current textbook of medicine, and you will find little attention or mention of the illness-words that concern patients. Words like *burden, stigma, waiting, loss* and *despair* are given little space in doctors' textbooks. We will address the topic of illness-words in Chapter 3.

MEDICINE'S MISNOMERS

One could forgive a profession some of its historic misnomers, were it not for the enormous number of such inaccuracies that persist, and the fact that modern practitioners of medicine aspire to the concept of individualised or precision medicine. In his 2015 State of the Union address, President Barack Obama announced the launch of the Precision

Medicine Initiative in the United States. Precision medicine has been driven by technical advances in medicine which enable more refined molecular diagnoses and identification of subsets of disease for which a distinct and specific therapy may be designed. This favours the 'splitters' within the medical profession, who seek subsets of patients with different forms of the same disease, over the 'lumpers', who try to see a bigger picture and seek commonalities across all patients. Precision medicine also demands the use of accurate terminology for disease description and classification; this will be a new challenge for medicine.

Every sub-speciality in medicine can produce an extensive list of misnomers or imprecise descriptions and terms for common conditions. For example, *biliary colic* is not a colic (a spasmodic or crampy pain that waxes and wanes), *pernicious anaemia* is no longer pernicious, *vitamin D* is more a hormone than a vitamin, and *autoimmune* diseases are immune-mediated but rarely '*auto*immune'. This is not merely a matter of semantics; one can readily see how imprecise terminology causes confusion and may promote imprecise thinking and poor medical judgement. Consider the example of chronic inflammatory bowel disease, the two main forms of which are ulcerative colitis and Crohn's disease, and for which the treatment differs. However, despite its name, ulcerative colitis doesn't ulcerate (except in very severe cases), whereas ulceration is the characteristic early feature of Crohn's disease.

A CROCKERY OF CROTCHETS

The word 'crotchet' can mean different things: a hook, a surgical instrument, a musical note, or a typographical punctuation when appearing as a pair, but everyone knows what *crotchety* means. Academics may be crotchety when they express highly individual and usually eccentric opinions or preferences for correct word usage. However, even non-academics have a short list of overused and abused words, phrases and expressions that represent irritants to be avoided. These are crotchets. Crotchets are generally harmless, of no practical importance, but in the health sciences, where language and communication must be effective, clear and precise, they assume greater importance.

Crotchets in medicine are difficult to eradicate, and they endure despite the efforts of several commentators who have recorded personal lists of the most irritating examples of bad medical language.[5] Crotchets tend to fall into various specific categories. First, there are the redundancies, such as the *past medical history*. If it's history, it's in the past. Similarly, *future progress, end result* and *track record* do not need to be two-word descriptors. Likewise, *skin rashes*: where else can a rash occur but on the skin!

Then, there are more troubling crotchets that estrange patients from their doctors because of obfuscation. These include the unnecessary use of big, unfamiliar and unnecessary words. For example, when the cause of a condition is known, doctors seem to have no difficulty making a positive declaration in simple language ('The cause of your cough is smoking'), but when there is uncertainty, they resort to unfamiliar words like *aetiology*, *essential* and *idiopathic*. Instead of saying 'We don't know the cause', there is aggrandisement – the implication being that this ignorance comes in spite of the fact that members of the medical profession are the rather grand bearers of enormous amounts of medical knowledge. When doctors cause disease or harm their patient, the result is referred to as *iatrogenic*.

Another form of language manipulation which qualifies as a crotchet is the creation of a verb by fusing the letters '*-ise*' or '*-ize*' with a noun. This may be acceptable for inanimate objects in an abstract way, but it has a distancing effect when applied to patients. Examples include: *digitalise* the patient (treat with the drug digitalis) and *hospitalise*. John Humphrys, in his book *Lost for Words,* on the mangling and manipulation of the English language, listed several egregious examples from daily life. However, he acknowledged that some experts on language, like David Crystal, feel that objecting to these neologisms is futile. Humphrys concedes that statements like 'Mr Patient was hospitalised' contain two less words than the alternative statement 'Mr Patient was admitted to hospital', but this is at the expense of removing something from Mr Patient, and from the hospital. Mr Patient has been transformed somehow by the first statement, but retains his identity in the second statement. At the same time, the hospital, which is a living place of caring, is reduced to an impersonal process in the first statement. Ironically, it is difficult to resist the use of words created by adding '*-ise*', as Humphrys notes, in claiming that the first statement above dehumanises and depersonalises Mr Patient. In a later chapter, we will see how Mr Patient, himself, may be a creation of words, and over-medicalised!

The most serious category of crotchet includes the recurring imprecisions. Common examples include: *the vital signs are stable* (not if you only measured them once); *the blood pressure is normal* (only the actual numbers suffice); and *the nervous system is grossly intact* (so, you didn't examine it). A variant of the last of these is *NAD: nothing abnormal detected* (nothing obvious).

CLICHÉS: SOMEONE ELSE'S PREJUDICE

The first cousins of the crotchets are the clichés. Clichés have been used extensively in medical textbooks as *aides-memoires*. However, blind adherence to these forms of borrowed wisdom can impede accurate diagnosis, cloud judgement and distort decision-making. To borrow from Oliver Wendell Holme's Jr: 'the minute a phrase becomes current, it becomes an apology for not thinking accurately'. Pity the poor patient with Parkinson's disease who has to wait for the doctor to witness a *festinating gait* before stumbling to the diagnosis. Even worse, is the notion that *fat, fertile and forty* might be a diagnostic profile for the bearer of gallstones. Although some of these jaded jingles now seem quaint, others, such as *coffee ground vomitus* (as sign of upper gut bleeding) and faeces that are *pale, foul and offensive* (steatorrhoea, or malabsorption of fat) are more difficult to dispel. Every day in our hospitals, innocent patients are subjected to unnecessary gastroscopies because nurses and junior doctors have learned in outdated textbooks that inspecting vomitus for anything reminiscent of 'coffee grounds' is an important diagnostic strategy. That may have had some significance when bleeding from duodenal ulceration was common, but today one is unlikely to learn much from searching for coffee grounds in vomitus, except in the odd patient who has ingested raw coffee grounds. Likewise, the term 'pale, foul and offensive' is probably more apt as a descriptor for certain politicians than as a diagnostic cue for malabsorption.

REFORMING THE MEDICAL RECORD

What's wrong with the following entry in a medical record?

> Mr White is a somewhat pleasant, Irish unemployed labourer and a known cirrhotic. He was hospitalised complaining of dysphagia [difficulty swallowing]. He has a history of angina but claims it has not been a problem lately. He denies smoking and admits to drinking three pints of beer each day.

In addition to the soft bigotry and stigmatising descriptors, (discussed later, in Chapter 7), this type of note distances the reader from the patient by translating the presenting symptom into medical-speak, by excluding the patient's voice, and by the unnecessary insertion of pejorative and perhaps prejudicial language. Patients don't *claim* anything. They state the facts as they know them, and they tend to tell the truth and do not need to *deny* or *admit* anything.

Reforming medical language is not easy. Several clinicians have suggested that this process should begin by reforming the medical record, medical case reports, and how doctors describe patients' problems to one another.[6] Sadly, this kind of reform has not been uniformly adopted. Simple recommendations, like giving the patient a voice in the record by including the patient's own description of the presenting problem, would be a good beginning. Instead, doctors tend to translate the patient's ordinary description of their symptoms into medical-speak, thereby frequently losing the essence of the problem. In almost all instances, the precise words first used by a patient to describe a symptom are the most valuable, and should be recorded before the description is corrupted by a clinician or triage nurse. For example, no one arrives at a doctor's office or at an emergency room complaining of angina pectoris or dysphagia. Contrary to what one might think, these fancy terms are interpretations, not direct translations, and are not necessarily more precise. The patient's *exact* words are more revealing: 'I have a sharp, jabbing pain' is quite different to 'I feel heaviness on my chest', and 'I experience a kind of fullness after eating, as if the food is getting stuck' is quite different to 'The food gets stuck while I'm eating and I can't get it down.' Once the patient's words have been recorded, further detail may then be obtained with open, or occasionally leading, questions as required.

The value of including the patient's voice in his or her own medical record not only enhances the accuracy of the record but may also provide insight into the significance and context of their symptoms. Symptoms come alive when the patient's account of what it means to be ill are included in the medical record. Doctors, nurses and other carers obviously need to pay attention to the stories patients have to tell. Humans think and communicate through stories. Moreover, storytelling is part of the coping and healing process. These simple truths are not new, but have become central to what has become known as narrative medicine. My interest here is not the theory of narrative medicine, some of which has been challenged.[7] Rather, my concern is the value of hearing and recording the patient's voice. For example, the patient's answers to the following simple questions suggested by Dr William J. Donnelly are usually highly informative, and should be part of the medical record: 'What is your understanding of your condition?' and 'How does your condition affect your life?'

The chronic illness of Charles Darwin is a historic example of the importance of the patient's words in reaching an accurate diagnosis and an understanding of suffering. Darwin's medical complaints have been a source of fascination for many, over the course of more than a century. (The renowned naturalist died in 1882.) On the one hand, are those who prefer to believe that Darwin suffered from some form of rare, obscure physical ailment, which perplexed his numerous doctors and from which the great man suffered in noble defiance. On the other, are the proponents of a psychosocial disorder, possibly hypochondria. When I studied Darwin's own words, recorded in his voluminous correspondence and in his diary, an obvious diagnosis emerged. Most illness-stories involve a weave of physical and psychological inputs, and Darwin's story was no different in that respect. It is likely that he had a common presentation with something ordinary, rather than an uncommon presentation with something extraordinary. Second-hand accounts of Darwin's symptoms have created a mystery, but Darwin's own words suggest that he had irritable bowel syndrome. The diagnosis of this condition is based only on a patient's symptoms, and Darwin left copious accounts of his symptoms – which require no contrived diagnoses. This was a common condition which can be disabling, and was suffered with great dignity by an extraordinary man.

THE BAD HISTORIAN

There is no such thing as a patient who is a *bad historian*. Bad histories are the handiwork of bad history-taking doctors. The way in which a patient provides a history is revealing in itself. Whether the history is succinct or hesitant, factual or vague, delivered anxiously or with jovial frivolity and throwaway remarks, it is always informative to a careful listener. The distinction between the fictional bad historian and the poor history-taker is well shown in the case of an elderly patient attending the emergency room. Up to one in every six elderly patients referred to the emergency department may have delirium. Delirium (acute disturbance of cognition or consciousness) is a neurologic emergency that requires no extraordinary expertise but is often missed when a patient is labelled as a 'bad historian'. In a commentary published in the *Journal of the American Medical Association,* Dr Des O'Neill despairingly noted that not once has he met a trainee doctor outside the speciality of geriatric medicine who correctly made the diagnosis of delirium. This, he attributed to the continued use of the term 'bad historian'.

SALUTATIONS, SLANG, CODES AND SECRET LANGUAGE

Language is not merely a tool for communication, it is also a reflection on how we think and practise. In short, the sloppiness of medical language may be a reflection on the contemporary status of caring. Therefore, concepts of what is acceptable or unacceptable change over time. No longer would words like *imbecile, idiot, mongol, lunatic, spastic, retard* and *cripple* ever be used to refer to a patient. However, equally distasteful words have emerged, which, if overheard, add to the burden of illness, create stigma, and may be deeply upsetting for families struggling to cope with a loved one's illness. These often pass as dark humour and are explained by apologists as a strategy for coping with professional stress.

What is wrong with the following modes of address for a person in crisis, whom carers may hardly know? 'My dear man, young lady, mate, Harry, grandpa'? Illness is difficult enough without casual, thoughtless and undignified language. Common sense should dictate that carers consciously evaluate at what stage in the relationship it is appropriate to switch from formality to familiarity. It is, of course, always possible to be kind and friendly while maintaining professional formality.

Ill-chosen words, technical terms and jargon are not the only linguistic problems that distance patients from their doctors. Doctors and nurses use codes and slang to describe certain kinds of patients in terms that they would not wish the patient to know about. Much of it has been popularised in television shows and in books like *The House of God*, which was written under the pen-name of Samuel Shem. More recently, comprehensive lists of medical slang have been assembled.[8] However, doctors have always used codes. The French have an expression for the worried-well patient who arrives with symptoms listed on a small piece of paper: *La maladie du petit papier*. The stereotype is a source of judgment bias, because such patients are erroneously thought to have no significant illness. The expression *heart-sink patient* is used to describe the patient who repeatedly returns to the clinic, and who is rarely satisfied. Usually, it is a patient with whom the doctor has not bonded. This is discussed later, in Chapter 8. The quirkiest code I have encountered was the one left by a colleague to signal to me that the patient being referred was, as others might uncharitably describe, *one sandwich short of a picnic,* or *not the sharpest tool in the box*. Rather than risk offending the patient, he simply placed on the referral letter the following notation, $11^{1/2}d$. To most people, this would go unnoticed, but to those of my generation in the British Isles, it refers to pre-decimalisation currency, meaning a halfpenny short of a shilling, or *not the full shilling*.[9] Of course, it is unacceptable to put anything offensive in a patient's chart. The chart should be considered the patient's property and, whether this document is handwritten or electronic, it should always be assumed that it will be read by third parties, and should always be self-explanatory.

ABBREVIATIONS

A friend sought my advice recently regarding an acute malady which required little more than analgesia and an antibiotic. When his concerned wife, a biochemist, asked if she could help, I reassured her that with a little 'TLC' (tender loving care) from her, he would recover promptly. *'Thin layer chromatography!'* she replied. 'How could that be of help?' Hard to believe, but even the most obvious or common abbreviation may have an alternative meaning, even in different parts of the same hospital. What a difference three letters can make. In a clever poem entitled 'Misunderstanding', Dr Eric Dyer recorded his misunderstanding upon reading 'Discontinue TLC' in a patient's chart, only later to discover that 'TLC', in this context, meant *triple lumen catheter* in the intensive care unit. When the stakes are high, nothing can be assumed.

Dr Bernard Lown describes a more serious instance of misunderstanding in his book *The Lost Art of Healing*. Lown recalls the case of a woman with long-standing TS (tricuspid stenosis, or narrowing of the tricuspid heart valve). When she overheard her doctor using the term 'TS' when discussing her medical problem with junior staff' she interpreted it to mean *terminal situation* – with tragic consequences.

Ambiguous abbreviations are still pervasive in medicine. Far from being expedient, they are a repeated source of miscommunication, medication errors and risk for patient safety. Non-conventional abbreviations have been outlawed by many regulatory authorities, and abbreviations which jeopardise patient safety have been well publicised. Medical records and communications among healthcare professionals have been remarkably resistant to the enforcement of policies designed to reduce the use of abbreviations. In one fatal case of missed hypercalcaemia (too much calcium in the blood) secondary to hyperparathyroidism (over-activity of the parathyroid gland), it was claimed unconvincingly that a chart-notation listing the abnormal numbers for calcium would have been overlooked because of abbreviated English words (Cal, Sod, Pot) instead of chemical symbols (eg. Ca^{++}, Na^+, K^+). Most clinicians can recall a similar case of a near-miss or tragic outcome in relation to the misinterpretation of laboratory results or drug dosages or frequency of administration, but the practice of abbreviating essential information seems to continue apace.

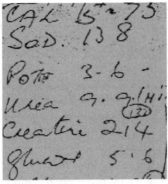

Mistaken abbreviations. A fatal case of missed hypercalcaemia actually had a clear notation of the abnormal calcium in the chart; the suggestion that one abbreviation (Ca^{++}) might be preferable to another (Cal) added insult to injury.[10]

NAME MY CONDITION

Comedians joke about the names doctors give to diseases. 'If I've got Barrett's, who's got mine?' Or, as Billy Connolly announced when he was diagnosed with Parkinson's disease: 'I wish he [Parkinson] had kept it to himself.' Eponyms in medicine are a legacy from an earlier time: they were once intended to honour the original discovery. However, in many cases they have outlived their purpose, and they are often inaccurate or misattributed. For example, Dr Burrill Crohn was alphabetically the first of three authors who, in 1932, described what is now known as Crohn's disease. The contribution of the other two is forgotten, but none of them deserved the credit, because the condition had been described by a Scottish surgeon, T. K. Dalziel, decades earlier, and probably earlier again by the Polish surgeon Antoni Leśniowski.

Some eponyms are tainted, and add insult to the injury suffered by patients.[11] For example, chronic inflammatory disorders such as Wegener's granulomatosis or Reiter's syndrome inadvertently celebrate the memory of alleged racists and Nazi sympathisers. It is difficult enough to be afflicted with such a disorder, without continuously being reminded that it honours the memory of such monsters.

Asperger's syndrome is the term first introduced by British child psychiatrist Dr Lorna Wing in 1981 to honour the work of the Austrian child psychiatrist Hans Asperger, for his concept of 'autistic psychopathy', which has since been subsumed under the term 'autism spectrum disorder'. At that time, neither Dr Wing nor her colleagues were aware of Hans Asperger's role in the Nazi killing regime which dispensed with children who were considered unfit for their ideal of the *volk*, a homogenous Aryan race. Although Asperger was not personally involved in the killing, and not a member of the Nazi Party, he was a conscious participant in a system of mass killing. These are the inescapable conclusions by investigative historians Herwig Czech and Edith Sheffer.[11] Dr Wing came to regret ever coining the Asperger eponym, and told Dr Adam Feinstein: 'I wish I hadn't done it. I would like to throw all labels away today, including "Asperger's syndrome". . . . Labels don't mean anything, because you get such a wide variety of profiles.'

Accuracy, even at the expense of brevity, is preferred in medicine, but a literary eponym is easily remembered, and can portray complex behaviours, with an economy of words, that are untainted, kinder and gentler, and unlikely to cause offense.

The Literary Alternative

There is a cartoon caption in one of Jim Unger's *Herman* series that I've always liked for its telling simplicity. A woman faces her doctor and says: 'I think we had much nicer diseases when I was a girl.' Once was a time when medicine was vaguely mystical and distant; now, it is harsh, real and fearsome. Would you prefer to have *obesity-hypoventilation syndrome* (OHS), as doctors now call it, or *Pickwickian syndrome,* as it was once known? Pickwickian syndrome is named after the character Joe from Charles Dickens' novel *The Pickwick Papers,* which has been beloved by generations since it first appeared in the early nineteenth century. Joe exhibited many of the symptoms later described by clinicians, including obesity and sleep apnoea (periodic absences of breathing during sleep).

Since doctors and writers each deal in stories of human experience, it is not surprising that many disorders, mostly psychological, have been inspired by figures in popular literature. The best known of all is perhaps the *Oedipus complex*, to describe a son's relationship with his mother. Many literary-inspired labels refer to a behaviour or psychological profile, and not necessarily to a pathological disorder. Examples include *Pollyanna syndrome* (from the Eleanor H. Porter children's heroine), an irritating friend who exhibits unrelenting or unrealistic optimism, or *Dorian Gray syndrome,* from the Oscar Wilde novel – and which might well summarise the modern-day obsession with youthful appearance.

Medicine has always drawn on literature to name anatomical structures and diseases. The *Achilles tendon* refers to the one vulnerability of the Greek hero Achilles, who was held by the heel when dipped as a child by his mother Thetis into the magically invulnerability-inducing waters of the River Styx. Likewise, the *atlas* vertebra relates to Atlas of Greek mythology, because it supports the globe of the skull. *Panic* is from the Greek god Pan, who instilled excessive or irrational fear in humans, whereas the literary origin of the word *syphilis* is more recent – from the Middle Ages, when the disorder was recognised. While the origin of the disease has always been in dispute, with each nation, country or ethnic group blaming another, the word was introduced by the Italian physician-poet Girolamo Fracastoro in 1530, in an epic poem in which a shepherd named Syphilus insulted Apollo for the parching effects of the sun – to which the deity responded by inflicting the dreaded disease.

Richard Asher first used the term *Munchausen syndrome* in 1951 to describe patients who fabricate illness and waste time and healthcare resources. The name is from Baron von Munchausen, an eighteenth-century German officer who told tall tales of his travels and travails. The paediatrician Roy Meadow later used the term *Munchausen syndrome by proxy* to refer to the deliberate fabrication of illness in relation to a child or other person being cared for by the person reporting the illness.

To illustrate the value of literary eponyms, my colleague Charlie Marks proposed that we write about a curious physical sign that is often seen in seriously ill patients who are delirious or terminally ill. Continual grasping at clothing or bed linen by the dying or delirious patient has been well recognised over the centuries. Anyone specialising in palliative and end-of-life care will be familiar with the observation, which usually signals that death is close. In today's medicalised society, most people die in hospitals or nursing homes, but earlier generations commonly witnessed death in the home, and were aware of this sign of imminent death. There are extensive references to the phenomenon in contemporary literature and portraiture, since most of the great artists and writers had something to say about life and death, doctors and diseases.

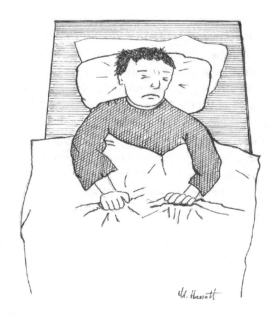

Gustave Flaubert gives an eloquent description of the sign as exhibited by Emma on her death bed in *Madam Bovary*, and Tolstoy was likewise explicit in his description of the death of Nikolai from tuberculosis in *Anna Karenina*. Similarly, the last person to attend to Marcel Proust recorded that he was clutching at the bedclothes, and recognised from 'peasant lore' that this was 'an infallible sign of the close and inevitable end'. Likewise, in Albert Camus's fictional account of a dying child in *The Plague*, 'His claw-like fingers were feebly plucking at the sides of the bed. Then they rose, scratched at the blanket over his knees and suddenly he doubled up his limbs, bringing his thighs above his stomach, and remained quite still.' Francisco Goya depicted the same sign in *Self-portrait with Dr. Arrieta* in 1820. Doubtless, there are countless other examples in literature and portraiture. Although the sign is well known to those familiar with death and dying, it has an ugly medical name, *carphology* (picking at bedclothes) and *floccilation* (picking at imaginary objects). However, four hundred years ago, Shakespeare wrote of the sign in *Henry V,* when Mistress Quickly announces the death of Falstaff after she observed him 'fumble with the sheets' and 'knew there was but one way'. Dr Charles Marks and I have proposed that the sign be known as *Henry V sign* and that the cacophonous medical terms should be abandoned. Advantages of a literary eponym, such as *Henry V sign*, include familiarity, ease of recall, the fact that it requires no specialist knowledge, and that its source is accessible to both the lay and medical community.

From the disease-focused language of doctor-speak, let us now move to the illness-words used by patients.

3

∽ઝ∽ઝ∽ઝ

The Illness Words

'I want to tell you how it feels. I want to explain it, to use my words.'
—Vivian Bearing in *W;t* by Marget Edson

*Hope – Suffering – Loss – Fear – Anger – Denial – Degradation – Shame
– Loneliness – Disbelief – Gain – Trust – Humour*

Serious illness strikes like violence. The routine of what we call health is abruptly shattered; 'in a minute a cannon batters all' is how John Donne described it on his sickbed. When we fall ill, we fall 'under the hard hand of science' and into the rift of its 'alien terminology', writes Anne Boyer. Boyer is a poet and essayist who was diagnosed with an aggressive form of breast cancer at the age of forty-one. In *The Undying*, her 2019 meditation on modern illness, she writes:

> To be declared with certainty ill while feeling with certainty fine is to fall on the hardness of language without being given an hour of soft uncertainty in which to steady oneself with preemptive worry.

In medical school, I learned about the disease-words used by doctors. I spent my career investigating the objective evidence of disease, in order to understand the mechanisms of disease. But there is another set of words used by patients that are seldom used in medical school, and never in the research laboratory – and which are curiously absent from textbooks of medicine. I would later learn from my patients the importance of using their words: the words that relate to their experiences and concerns. These words need attention and deliberation. These are the illness-words.

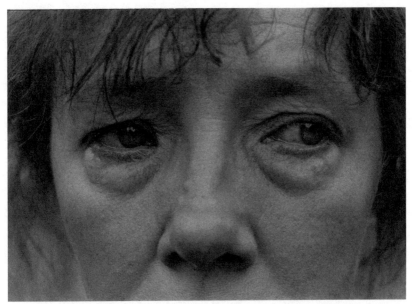

Illness Face Detail of Jo Spence/Terry Dennett
© *Jo Spence Memorial Archive, Ryerson Image Centre. Reproduced by permission.*

HOPE

Faced with the prospect of giving up or continuing, hope is what propels us forward. Considered a necessary trait for a successful life, hope has been defined by Alisdair MacIntyre as a 'belief in a reality that transcends what is available as evidence'. Hope is at the heart of what it means to be human. It is one of the theological virtues, integral to the ascent of man. Whereas despair seems easy and impatient, and looks to the past with certainty, hope is hard working, looks to the future and is full of uncertainty.

Hope has fascinated poets and philosophers through the ages. Alexander Pope's 'Hope springs eternal in the human breast' from *An Essay on Man,* remains both poetic, and a profound nod to human potential and possibility. For Emily Dickinson (1830-86), 'hope is the thing with feathers'; in an extended metaphor, she transformed hope into a feathered bird permanently perched within all humans, always there to help us, never asking anything of us, except that we live our lives as fully as possible. Of course, like all living things, hope is both resilient and fragile; it is part of our humanity, but not to be taken for granted.

Rebecca Solnit has reflected on historical stories with wonderful possibilities, to find hope and optimism for the future in an uncertain world. Extraordinary achievements by ordinary people, either alone or in collaboration with others, are inspirational. At all times, there is uncertainty, and the object of hope is not always obvious. In a tribute to a failed rebellion by a band of Irish peasants against unspeakable imperial oppression, the poet Seamus Heaney described a pathetic scene where 'terraced thousands died, shaking scythes at cannon'. Seemingly engaged in a hopeless cause, against impossible odds, the peasants, with 'pockets of our greatcoats full of barley', were crushed, 'the hillside blushed' with their bloodshed. They were buried 'without shroud or coffin', but hope remained, because 'in August the barley grew up out of the grave'. Another generation would follow, inspired to complete the struggle.

The portrayal of *Hope* by G. F. Watts at Tate Britain in London illustrates the importance of the phenomenon. This influential image, of a blindfolded woman astride a globe, playing a tune on a damaged instrument with a single string, after all the others have snapped, is a subtle, enigmatic and compelling symbol of perseverance even when all seems lost. The portrait has influenced religious and political leaders, and provided inspiration for what has popularly become known as the 'audacity of hope'.

Every doctor has stories to tell of patients who deteriorated once hope was lost, or when hope was removed by an insensitively delivered comment or opinion from another healthcare worker. Likewise, most doctors have been impressed with how hope can energise a patient. Most recall different patients with the same condition, or at the same clinical stage of disease, but with divergent outcomes, seemingly because of differences in the degree of hope on the part of the patient.

There is an important distinction between avoiding giving false hope, on the one hand, and actively removing a patient's hope, on the other. The famous physician, William Osler, warned his peers: 'It is not for you to don the black cap and assuming the judicial function, take hope away from any patient'. Another physician, Hacib Aoun,[1] who was, himself, diagnosed with a serious illness, invoked his colleagues to consider that the 'fewer the therapeutic options available, the greater the involvement with the patient should be'. Moreover, 'Hope is the one thing that even if we cannot push ourselves as physicians to provide, we should at the very least not deny . . . I, of course, do not mean that we must provide false assurances, but you must let them know that if there is a chance, however small, that you will pursue it and that you won't give up on the patient. You will always be on their side.'

Hope is often balanced against realism, but the two can co-exist. Deception need not be a tipping-point. Hope does not mean denying realities. Hope can be calibrated. When there is no chance of cure, hope can still exist for the quality of time that remains. In a story beautifully told by Dr Alexandra (Sandy) Levine, a young man was diagnosed with an aggressive form of cancer and was offered the hope of multiple-drug chemotherapy, on the understanding that some patients had benefited from such treatment. He accepted the treatment, but after just one year, he died. Years later, the young man's mother remained grateful to Dr Levine, because the doctor's treatment had allowed her son to 'to live that year instead of dying that year'. In his mother's view, hope transformed the remainder of her son's short life from one of dying to a time of living.

With sensitive language, a physician can guide a patient to calibrate hope from cure to comfort. The chance to die at home, to be with loved ones, and not to be alone, may be sufficient grounds for hope for many.

In a memoir under the curious title *The Cost of Hope*, the award-winning journalist Amanda Bennett raised disturbing questions about the extraordinary cost of medical treatments for a serious illness in America when the outcome is uncertain. The book tells the story of her beloved husband's diagnosis with a rare form of kidney cancer, and their seven-year quest to buy time to extend his life. Was it necessary to spend over $600,000 and undergo seventy-six CT scans? She emphatically declares that their struggle was better than conceding defeat, and that given the chance, she would do it again. The 'cost of our hope was good for us'. She questions her own motives, and whether it was all for her husband or, in part, for herself. Could things have been done differently? Most of her questions are unanswerable. The cost of the fight for life was, she says, 'so much more than I believe it should have, and that expense put that hope far beyond the reach of too many others'. She writes of love and loss, but in the end, the inescapable conclusion is that while the cost of medical interventions may be quantifiable, hope, like love and life, has no price.

John Betjeman's poem 'Devonshire Street W.1' snatches out of time an ordinary moment following a diagnosis of terminal illness. An ordinary scene: an ordinary couple leaves the doctor's consulting rooms. No doubt about the diagnosis: conclusive. ('The heavy mahogany door with its wrought-iron screen/ Shuts.') Devonshire Street is a real place not far from Harley Street. 'No hope.' With the X-rays tucked under his arm, the patient and his wife stand alone, but life outside goes on: 'the sun still shines on . . . merciless, hurrying Londoners!' Although the door shuts (nothing more to be done) and life goes on, the patient is not alone. He is accompanied by his wife ('She puts her fingers in his'), as a loving ally who reminds him of past times, and how he still has their marriage to help him cope. It is their marriage and memories that are now more important than the news of his terminal illness. The poem resonates with a short story told by the palliative-care specialist Frank Brennan, who describes a woman determined to honour her marriage vow – 'till death do us part' – and remain with her dying husband. The hope they had was for the time they had left. And that is always worth something.

Hope is neither expectancy nor anticipation, and not necessarily the prospect of resolution of all that is amiss, or much that is tangible, but hope does look toward the prospect of something better. One thing seems clear: the other side of hope is despair, and that makes the suffering of illness greater.

SUFFERING

Relief of suffering is central to the mission of all healthcare organisations, and yet, *suffering* is a word seldom seen in patients' records or spoken by doctors. Curiously, the term is explicitly discouraged in medical texts, along with other words that describe patients as victims. Convention prefers that patients be recorded as *having* symptoms and complications rather than actually *suffering* from them! Why? In a 2013 article, one physician concluded that doctors avoid the word 'suffering' because it is so varied and because it is not 'actionable' – meaning that doctors frequently don't know how to deal with it when its cause is not obvious.[2] While there are insurance reimbursement codes and drugs for pain and anxiety, there are none for suffering. The relief of suffering calls for something that may lie beyond the capacity of what most doctors can offer.

Chronic suffering has become more common with the rise of chronic disease, and because medical advances prolong illness by keeping patients alive. However, suffering is no longer considered ennobling or spiritually fortifying. Religious perspectives on suffering have largely been eclipsed by a more common view that suffering is pointless and unnecessary, and amenable to medical technology. Pointless or otherwise, it is core to human experience to seek a meaning for suffering. The philosopher Scott Samuelson has found seven ways of looking at 'pointless suffering' while acknowledging an immense paradox of human life: to be human is to accept and reject suffering simultaneously. In other words, suffering represents the gap between how the world is, and how we think it should be.

In a landmark article almost thirty years ago, 'The Nature of Suffering and the Goals of Medicine', published in the *New England Journal of Medicine*, and later in his book of the same title, Dr Eric Cassell described suffering as 'an affliction of the *person*, not the body'. Cassell defined suffering as 'the state of severe distress associated with events that threatens the intactness of person'. It is, he says, 'the increasing awareness of the impact of the physical state on the person, not the physical impairments per se, that causes suffering.' This calls for a rejection of the traditional mind/body dualism: mind and body are inseparable. Separating disease from the person – the personal suffering – is one of the failings of modern medicine. Treatment of disease alone, even when delivered with kindness and compassion, often fails to relieve suffering. Consider the person who experiences an acute neurological injury from a stroke; recovery of function is not tantamount to relief of suffering if he or she is left with fear of the unknown, loss of earning capacity due to the inability to drive, for example, and loss of confidence and security. Suffering is not confined to the physical symptoms associated with stroke, and it may go undetected unless the patient is asked about it directly.

When Cassell asked patients whether they were suffering, they were often quizzical, unsure of what he meant. Clues to the source of their suffering lay beyond the confines of the physical entity of their disease. Close questioning and close listening was required. For some, words fail to express adequately the level of suffering. In recalling King Lear's suffering as he carried the corpse of Cordelia, the surgeon and author Richard Selzer commented: 'The symptom of suffering lies outside the precinct of language. It cannot be rendered. In such moments, only howled vowels will do.' Too often, however, it is borne silently.

'I'm learning to suffer' remarks the fictional Vivian Bearing. As the doctors focus on her disease, her distress is complex due not solely to her physical disease and its treatment, but also to her disturbed sense of self. Drugs and medical technology can relieve suffering from physical symptoms such as pain, but for other forms of suffering, engagement with the person, rather than the disease, is required. This engagement begins with acknowledgement of the suffering: bearing witness, and a commitment not to abandon the patient. In the words of Dr Hacib Aoun, 'when there is no cure, there is still much to be done to alleviate suffering'.

Cassell's classic description of human suffering has not gone completely unchallenged: others have tried to capture the concept of suffering with more ordinary, accessible language. 'Soul pain' is how Dr Michael Kearney, an Irish palliative-care expert, describes human suffering. For others, the two essential elements of suffering which distinguish it from superficial or transient emotional states are a lasting negative affective experience (persisting mood disturbance) and a loss of a person's sense of self.[4]

Loss

Illness is all about loss: loss of control, of function, of confidence, of occupation, of income, of identity, of future and, in some cases, of hope. 'I have never forgotten the sense of powerlessness . . . . You are in someone else's hands . . . the patient is never in charge', writes the essayist Sinéad Gleeson, describing her memories of arthritis in childhood and leukaemia in early adulthood. For historian Tony Judt, writing of his sense of imprisonment at night with motor neurone disease: 'helplessness is humiliating'.

As varied as the lived experience of illness is, the loss is never the same even for people with the same affliction. For Christopher Hitchens, famed for quick-wittedness as a conversationalist and debater, the loss of his voice to cancer was the cruellest blow. His hope, if not for a cure, was for remission. What he wanted back was 'in the most beautiful apposition of two of the simplest words in our language: the freedom of speech'.

For the philosopher Havi Carel, who developed a rare progressive lung disorder, the harshest of all was the loss of friends: 'friends who stay away because they do not know what to say'. Illness creates a new social barrier – and social isolation for the patient. Awkwardness in the presence of a sick person creates a distance, and drives away some colleagues and acquaintances. It also discourages the person afflicted with illness from participating in social encounters with strangers – thereby increasing their sense of isolation.

Carel also describes illness as a transformative experience – a struggle, in which the stakes are high. Recalling the Hans Christian Andersen story 'The Shadow', in which a man is subsumed by his shadow, Carel suggests that the shadow is life lived in the shadow of illness, and that, like the shadow, illness attempts to steal an identity and take, or take over, a life. When faced with the prospect of a lung transplant, the loss of identity is more manifest. Will she be the same person, she wonders? The transplant is more than an organ: it becomes a metaphor for a new identity, and a 'whole set of uncertainties, anxieties and concerns'.

Others have emphasised the transformative nature of illness. In Tolstoy's story 'The Death of Ivan Ilyich', when Ivan compares his image in a portrait with what he sees in the mirror, the physical change is profound, but Ivan is also forever changed psychologically. Reynolds Price captured the changing effect of serious illness in the title of his book *A Whole New Life,* written after he was diagnosed with a spinal cancer. From his experience, he was clear about the advice he would give to anyone confronted with a grave illness. First, 'You're in your present calamity alone, far as this life goes.' Second, generous people will wish to help, but will not be able to restore your main want, which is to recover 'the person you used to be'. Third, accept that you are 'not that person now', grieve for a limited time for whatever you have lost, and then 'find your way to be somebody else, the next viable you – a stripped-down whole other clear-eyed person, realistic as a sawed-off shotgun and thankful for air, not to speak of the human kindness you'll meet if you get normal luck'.

In *My Year Off: Rediscovering Life after a Stroke,* the literary critic Robert McCrum, while recovering, lamented the loss of his body parts, which merged with the added sense of loss of identity. He recorded in his diary: 'My image of myself these days has been of a beetle or cockroach without a leg, flailing helplessly and covered in dirt, on the brink of extinction.' Similarly, Oliver Sacks, the famous physician and author, described an unsettling distortion of body-image while in hospital for treatment of a leg injury (*A Leg to Stand On*). In addition to loss of sensation in the leg, he had a sense of loss of the leg belonging to him. Even more exasperating was the failure of his carers to acknowledge this problem. Although Sacks was aware that his lesion was a peripheral neurological one, he had acquired a sense that it had become central: 'not just a lesion in my muscle, but a lesion in me'. The disruption of his sense of self, which was far greater than would have been suggested by the paralysis and loss of sensation, persisted until he was able to walk again without thinking.

Loss of a sense of self, or identity, is common with all forms of illness, and is reflected in daily speech ('I'm not myself'). Likewise, carers often comment: 'She's not herself today'. However, the distress caused by this form of loss is an under-appreciated element of the suffering associated with illness.[5] The playwright Alan Bennett humorously captured the concept in *The Madness of George III,* in which the Queen complains that the doctors do not understand the King's intermittent madness because they don't really know him: 'It is the same with all the doctors. None of them know him. He is not himself. So how can they restore him to his proper self, not knowing what that self is?' In contrast to the doctors, the king has insight. ('I fear I am not in my perfect mind. Do not laugh at me.' When a well-wisher comments 'Your Majesty seems more yourself', he wittily replies: 'Do I? Yes, I do. I have always been myself, even when I was ill. Only now I *seem* myself. That's the important thing. I have remembered how to seem.'

Well-wishers seldom appreciate the degree of suffering of an ill person due to what has been lost. 'The best-meaning and most generously thoughtful friend or relative cannot hope to understand', according to Tony Judt, who dismissed 'well-meaning encouragements to find nonphysical compensations for physical inadequacy', and for what he had lost due to motor neurone disease. 'Loss is loss,' he wrote, 'and nothing is gained by calling it by a nicer name.'

FEAR

Fear is a commonly used word – but not by doctors. *Anxiety* is the word more commonly used by doctors. Although anxiety often accompanies fear, the two feelings are not synonymous. Whereas fear is an appropriate physiological 'fight-or-flight' response to anything that may threaten the physical integrity of an individual, anxiety is overlapping, but has additional causes and is often more prolonged. Drugs may relieve anxiety in a non-specific way, but the cause of fear needs to be directly addressed.

In her comprehensive *Fear: A Cultural History,* Joanna Bourke records that the nature of fear of death has changed over time. Fear of the unknown, strife or apocalyptic disasters has given way to fear of dying rather than fear of death itself. In the past, dying was fast and certain. Today it is more prolonged, modified by medical possibilities – which have changed but not defused the fear itself.

Fear is probably the most common emotion experienced by patients: fear of the unknown, of threat posed by illness, of loss of control, of what the doctor may say, of the harsh language of medicine, and of the dying process. For those who heal, there is fear of relapse. In some cases, there is fear of the truth being withheld. While undergoing treatment for a spinal cancer, the celebrated American author Reynolds Price asked himself: 'Why could I never tell my doctors the depth of my fear?' Patients in hospital talk among themselves about matters that they would never discuss with their doctors.

Fear is common to all patients, regardless of their level of education, and regardless of whether they are able to voice their fear. In some cases, patients may not be aware of their fear. Those who remain fearful tend to fare less well than those who are comforted and put at ease. Time spent with patients to inform, explain, reassure and put them at ease is rewarding, and most experienced clinicians can recall patients who experience objective improvements once fear subsides following reassurance and explanation.[1] Failure to address a patient's fears is a missed opportunity. Dr Michael Balint describes a patient's fears as an important 'opportunity for the doctor's therapeutic skill', particularly because dealing with fear belongs to the 'domain of common-sense therapy'.[2]

ANGER

'Why me?' 'Why *not* me!' 'Why not someone else?' 'Life is so unfair.' Anger burns those who become ill, the elderly as well as the rebellious adolescent, and they don't always know why they are angry. In some cases, anger is caused by illness itself, such as in dementia or other mental illnesses. Doctors, caregivers and loved ones often bear the brunt of the anger. In other cases, rage sustains an ability to stay in the mainstream of life. There is no shortage of illness-stories expressing anger with poor standards of care, and a desire to expose the outrages of modern medicine. Social psychologist Dr Carol Tavris argues in her book *Anger: The Misunderstood Emotion* that clinicians often take a simplistic approach to anger. Anger, she feels, should not be dismissed as a useless emotion that needs to be managed. Rather, it may have its uses, but first it needs to be understood as it is experienced, in different ways by different individuals. Depression, she says, 'is not anger turned inward; if anything, anger is depression turned outward. Follow the trail of anger inward, and there you find the small, still voice of pain.'

Loss of function, loss of control, loneliness, suffering, and a sense of unfairness, provides a background for anger to foment. This is often compounded by fatigue, stress, and frustrating delays, waiting for what may seem to be an uncaring health service. Then there are the tedious stories told by visitors who cannot sit still and listen, and the irritation of an endless supply of cheerfully offered advice: 'Cheer up', 'Don't be so negative', 'Be positive'. The tyranny of having to maintain a positive attitude is discussed elsewhere in this book (in Chapter 8).

Barbara Ehrenreich rails against the assumption that positive thinking is inherently good. Her prose seethes with anger and resentment at 'exhortations to think positively – to see the glass half full, even when it lies shattered on the floor'. The pervasiveness of this 'cult of cheerfulness' in self-help literature, popular psychology and upbeat illness-memoirs has, she contests, fooled modern society and increased the burden of illness, and continues to damage vulnerable patients, who feel obliged to suppress negative emotions when crisis strikes. The unfairness and added burden of fear caused by misleading positivism is sadly reflected in one patient's thoughts about personal responsibility:[6] 'I know I have to be positive all the time. . . . I know that if I get sad, or scared or upset, I am making my tumour grow faster and I will have shortened my life.' Ehrenreich was spared this additional burden when she was afflicted with breast cancer, because her 'persistent anger' shielded her. Similarly, Ann Boyer's prose seethes with anger in *The Undying: A Meditation on Modern Illness*:

> The world is blood pink with respectability politics, as if anyone who dies from breast cancer had died of a bad attitude or eating a sausage or not trusting the word of a junior oncologist. After my chemotherapy seems to work, people say how they knew that I, of course, would survive, as if I were someone so special and strong and all the others weren't.

Rage is variably expressed or suppressed by the ill. It is the language of the powerless. Silent rage is expressed in the images of Jo Spence as she recorded the stages of her illness and impending death from cancer. In a series of photographic self-portraits, Spence was determined to look at life, and illness, on her own terms. Her photographs depict the physical impact of breast cancer and its disfiguring treatment on her body. However, they represent a defiant ownership, a reclaiming of her body-image to the very end.

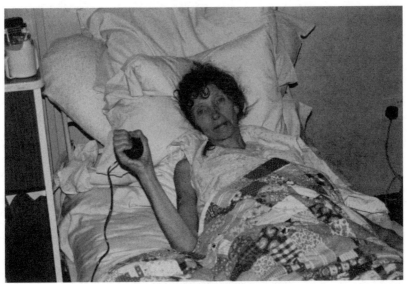

Jo Spence in a hospice bed
© *Jo Spence Memorial Archive, Ryerson Image Centre. Reproduced by permission.*

The short-story writer Lorrie Moore has captured the suppressed rage experienced by many parents dealing with a seriously ill child. In her desperation to cope with her child's cancer, a mother's thoughts race and rage: 'What nightmare this is. Is this all really happening?' Easily irritated by 'chirpy voices' and the 'airy scripted optimism' of well-meaning nurses, she is also intolerant of the notion of medicine as an inexact science or an art: 'if we wanted art, Doc, we'd go to an art museum'. She rejects hollow encouragement in order to adopt a positive attitude: 'Take a positive attitude. *Take a hike!*'

Dylan Thomas's poem 'Do not go gentle into that good night' acknowledges the transience of human existence and the inevitability of death, and famously invokes his father to cling to life as long as possible and to 'rage, rage against the dying of the light'. This is a different kind of rage from that expressed by Philip Larkin in his poem 'The Old Fools', which rages against the humiliations of growing old. Larkin presents an angry catalogue of harsh questions reflecting his horror, as his mother's personality slips away as a result of dementia. There is little room to rage, rage against the dying of the light here. In anticipation of his own end of life, and what it will feel like to experience 'the whole hideous inverted childhood', the poet's mood shifts from anger toward resignation: 'Well, we shall find out.'

In his autobiography, *Meaning of Disability*, Albert B. Robillard, a university professor of sociology who became paralysed in midlife with motor neurone disease, presents his illness and disability as if he were a living laboratory. The attention to detail is that of a trained observer. Anger, which is accorded a separate chapter, predominates, not only because of Robillard's loss of mobility but mainly because of difficulties with communication when his speech fails. His intended words and meanings are incorrectly translated, and repeatedly distorted, by carers. He becomes expert in anger and isolation, as he copes with the challenge of maintaining his identity.

Best-selling author Terry Pratchett, never one to go gentle anywhere, or into any night, was white with anger, 'a non-directional ball of fury', when he was diagnosed with a variant of early-onset Alzheimer's disease (posterior cortical atrophy). According to his friend Neil Gaiman, 'there is a fury to Terry Pratchett's writing. . . . The anger is always there, an engine that drives.' Anger was the driver for Pratchett's sense of what is fair and what is not. After his diagnosis, his anger was directed at his brain, the name of the disease, the health service and the 'unnecessary suffering' imposed by a country that refused people the right to decide the time and nature of their death. 'Days of Rage' is the subtitle for the final segment of a collection of Terry's reflections on his life and death. He regarded his Alzheimer's as 'an insult'. 'When in *Paradise Lost* Milton's Satan stood in the pit of Hell and raged at the Heaven, he was merely a trifle miffed compared to how I felt that day' – when he was diagnosed. 'You could have used my anger to weld steel.' And so he directed his anger in a constructive way against the disease. This included providing financial support for research and his efforts to increase awareness of the condition. For Pratchett, the first element of any strategy is to break down stigma, and to name, and speak about, the condition.

DENIAL

'Don't deny the diagnosis, defy the verdict' was a mantra of Norman Cousins, author and patient advocate. Denial is a label that presents a healthcare perspective rather than a patient's experience. It is judgemental, loaded with negative connotations, and linked with unhealthy behaviours such as non-adherence to medical advice. Denial is the first stage in Elizabeth Kübler-Ross's concept of progression during a serious illness, from denial to rage, and through bargaining to depression, and eventual acceptance. However, the model is open to challenge because it creates stereotypes and reduces complex human emotions to stages, which are actually overlapping. Moreover, denial is not always bad, nor is acceptance always desirable. Denial reflects (and deflects) the distress and suffering caused by illness. It should be considered as part of the complex process of adjusting to the change imposed by chronic illness. The enormous effort that patients invest in trying to appear 'normal' in public is under-appreciated: this 'tension between the private self and public identity' is part of the burden of illness and disability.[7] It should, therefore, not be surprising that some patients decline the role of 'good patient' and prioritise their own needs over the expectations of others. For many patients, denial has value as a temporary coping mechanism, a shield from the harsh immediacy of a diagnosis of serious illness.

Denial and concealment overlap but are not synonymous. Throughout history, political leaders and their minders have taken extraordinary measures to hide evidence of physical illness. This has been particularly well documented with several American presidents.[8] The case of Woodrow Wilson, twenty-eighth president (from 1913 to 1921), is particularly informative because it shows the profound influence of the context of illness on the form and degree of denial. Wilson's denial of his illness was studied by neuropsychiatrist Edwin A. Weinstein, who linked it with the president's pre-morbid personality, status in society, personal attitudes to work and accomplishment, and prevailing religious and cultural values. The most serious of Wilson's many illnesses was a series of strokes, the first at the age of thirty-nine, with recurrences during his presidency. Wilson's strict Protestant background has been linked with his view that becoming ill represented a moral weakness or dereliction of duty. According to Weinstein, 'denial became a means to avoid anxiety and depression and to preserve one's sense of personal integrity'. Like many others who are heavily work-oriented, often the leaders within a family, Wilson denied or minimised his disabilities. Weinstein points out that, 'like Wilson, patients are apt to refer to a disabled part of the body not as "my eye" or "my arm", but rather as "the eye" or "that arm".' To minimise his physical disability, he used euphemisms like *lame* rather than *paralysis*. Whatever the personal benefits of this form of denial, which was supported by his wife and physician, Wilson's illness-denial had international political implications, by influencing his attitudes and language, and the rhetoric of his public speeches.

Of course, denial may take different forms. Reluctance to accept personal responsibility for illness is often evident in the words patients use: 'My liver couldn't cope with the drink'; 'It was the drugs that made me do it'; 'I wasn't given enough tablets, so I stopped taking them'; 'I wasn't sent an appointment, so I didn't follow up'. In response, doctors need a language that is more direct than confrontational, more truthful than technical, and designed to help patients defy rather than deny illness.

Denial of illness is not exclusive to patients; it also occurs at societal and professional levels. One of the many paradoxes related to illness is how modern society tries to hide what is, in fact, a normal part of human life. In *The Illness Narratives*, Dr Arthur Kleinman writes: 'Images of widespread chronic illness are not what capitalist or socialist ideologies want to represent to their members as the states try to encourage consumption or mobilise enthusiasm for governmental campaigns. The imagery of infirmity and disorder provokes moral questions that most social systems prefer not to encourage.'

More than one hundred years ago, Tolstoy showed the harm caused by denial in *The Death of Ivan Ilyich*:

> Ivan Ilyich's chief torment was the lie – the lie that was for some reason acknowledged by all – that he was only ill, and was not dying, and that he only needed to keep calm and undergo treatment, and then something very good would come of it. Yet he knew that whatever they did, nothing would come of it, except for even more torturous suffering and death. And he was tormented by the lie, tormented by the fact that they did not want to admit what everyone knew, and what he knew, but wanted to lie . . . and they wanted him, forced him to take part in this lie himself.

The consequence of the lie was that Ivan Ilyich was deprived of pity and understanding, and at times felt ashamed. 'He wanted to be cuddled, kissed, cried over, as children are cuddled and comforted.'

Denial is also implicit when illness-memoirs present the outcome of serious illness or disease as a triumph. Anne Hunsaker Hawkins has analysed the myths underlying many illness-stories; these myths include rebirth, battle, journey, and what she refers to as 'the myth of healthy-mindedness'. The psychotherapist, and author of her own illness-memoir, Kathlyn Conway uses the term *triumph narrative* to challenge the myth of the beautiful sufferer who courageously beats illness and shares the lessons learned, emphasising positive thinking for others. Conway illustrates how the denial implicit in attempting to live out a triumph narrative, conforming with what others in society find desirable, may actually deprive patients of the means to cope better. For example, the determination of a blind individual to appear 'normal' not only puts him in danger but also deprives him of a walking-cane and visual aids which could have provided a greater degree of independence. Well-meaning parents may also become unwitting accomplices in the denial by rejecting special schools to protect the ill or disabled from becoming marginalised.

The medical and nursing professions have, in the past, frequently colluded in denial or obscuring the facts of illness. For this, they have been open to criticism of dishonouring the principle of truth-telling. In Simone de Beauvoir's memoir of her mother's illness and final weeks, the author and philosopher expresses regret for being complicit in a conspiracy of silence, a betrayal. First published in 1964, *A Very Easy Death* appeared before the modern era of palliative-care medicine. At no stage was her diagnosis or prognosis discussed with her mother by the doctors. While family and friends followed their lead, de Beauvoir was distressed with 'all this odious deception!' Too late, she could see the value of openness, and the damage caused to her mother by the silence: 'the truth was crushing her [Maman] and when she needed to escape from it by talking, we were condemning her to silence'.

Since the publication of *A Very Easy Death*, attitudes to truth-telling have changed considerably, but the notion of an 'easy death', and overt denial of the fact that the patient is ill, persists. In Le Ann Schreiber's 1990 account of her mother's illness with pancreatic cancer, *Midstream*, everyone appears to be in denial, including her ill mother. This, Schreiber writes, was caused, in part, 'because the doctors at the medical center continually misled her', and then everyone became complicit.

It often seems easier to flee from the truth than to face it, and defuse it. For the caregiver, this approach is convenient, not considerate. It is a selfish avoidance. 'But we had no choice: hope was her [Maman's] most urgent need', according to de Beauvoir. Hope is not the opposite of denial; hope can co-exist with truth when it is measured and proportionate. When disclosure of the facts of illness includes uncertainty about the future, there is room for hope.

DEGRADATION AND SHAME

Embarrassment, shame and humiliation feature in many illness-stories, and are particularly evident in the stories of doctors who have become patients. Dr Oliver Sacks described the 'systematic depersonalisation which goes with becoming-a-patient' in *A Leg To Stand On*, his account of a leg injury which was sustained while climbing in Norway but attended to in an English hospital. The 'grotesqueries' and 'dragged-out formalities' of hospitalisation were akin to being processed for entry to prison. Transformation from person to patient follows a ritual in which personal clothing is replaced with an anonymous hospital gown, the person's wrist is clasped by an identification bracelet, and their name is accompanied by a number. Conceding the need for institutional regulations, Sacks observed: 'One is no longer a person – one is now an inmate.'

While the degradations of the physical examination, with pokes, probes and prods, have provided rich material for stand-up comics, there are unspeakable humiliations for vulnerable individuals. Margaret Edson's fictional Vivian Bearing is a teacher who, after a series of degradations, including 'the agony of a proctosigmoidoscopy' [an internal examination of the bowel by insertion of a telescope-like instrument through the anus], 'watching myself go bald', and violent vomiting as a result of chemotherapy, is subjected to a pelvic examination by a junior doctor who was once one of her students.

Sinéad Gleeson's *Constellations* describes the experiences of a teenager with chronic arthritis of the hip, beset with a limp, surgical scars and asymmetry of her body. Schooldays were replaced with time in hospitals for investigations and surgery. Being self-conscious and different from other adolescents was bad enough, but the insensitivity of hospital staff, and their impatience with her reluctance to expose her body for terrifying investigations accentuated the mortification: 'I was a self-conscious girl being humiliated for her shame.' The 'doctor-patient relationship has its own imbalances . . . Every orthopaedic doctor who examined me during those years was male.'

Shame is the other side of stigma – and is often linked with a feeling of guilt. As we will see in Chapter 7, stigma is created by the response of others to one's illness, whereas shame is what one feels in the face of stigma. For doctors, shame is what accompanies their errors; for patients, by contrast, shame is the lived experience of stigma.

In his memoir, the author John Updike discusses his experience with recurrent episodes of psoriasis under the title *At War with My Skin*, in which he repeatedly uses the word 'shame'. Elsewhere, in the short story 'From the Journal of a Leper', he likens the condition to leprosy: 'The name of the disease, spiritually speaking, is Humiliation.' As a child, the author didn't learn to swim, because of his naked appearance; at school, an older boy asked if his rash was syphilis, but later his skin disease was enough to save him from being included in the military draft. Curiously, Updike concedes that humiliation was not entirely due to the reaction of others: 'my war with my skin had to do with self-love, with finding myself acceptable, whether others did or not.'

Lucy Grealy's *Autobiography of a Face,* published in 1994, is the story of a life dominated by her face, which was disfigured by cancer in childhood and then by the treatment for the cancer: 'I *was* my face. I *was* ugliness.' Born in 1963, Grealy and her family moved to the United States from Dublin when she was four. When she was nine, she was diagnosed with Ewing's sarcoma, an aggressive form of cancer. This required removal of a portion of her jaw, chemotherapy and radiotherapy; to restore her once-pretty face, she underwent thirty reconstructive operations, most of which were unsuccessful. She died, aged thirty-nine, from a drug overdose. Shame is what Lucy recalls when other children looked at her face: 'The cruelty of children is immense, almost startling in its precision.' Through the response of others to her face, she learned 'the language of paranoia: every whisper I heard was a comment about the way I looked, every laugh a joke at my expense'. Later, came taunts like 'dog girl'. Her account of her schooldays is direct and unsentimental, but nonetheless heart-rending: 'When my face gets fixed, then I'll start living.' Humiliated and exposed, is how she felt during a consultation with an oncologist.

In adulthood, Grealy realised the essence of stigma: it was others who were 'uncomfortable because of my face'. She had spent 'years being treated for nothing other than looking different from everyone else'. 'Beauty, as defined by society at large, seemed to be only about who was best at looking like everyone else.' The pain she felt as a result of feeling ugly was, she believed, the tragedy of her life: 'The fact that I had cancer seemed minor in comparison.'

In a remarkable sequel to Grealy's story, Thomas Couser, a professor of English, and expert on the illness-memoir genre, argued that her obituary, published in the *New York Times,* was 'a particularly ironic example of death writing inflicting posthumous harm', and that it heaped further stigma on its subject. The obituary implied that Grealy's death was by suicide, whereas her sister Suellan said it was the result of an accidental drug overdose. Couser correctly points out that Grealy's life is 'gravely diminished by its simplistic representation'. For example, the formulaic portrayal of Lucy's story as a triumph against adversity (but ultimately a failure), 'represents disability as a personal tragedy rather than as a social and cultural construct, removing stigma from the overcomer but not from the condition in question'. Like the well-meaning obituary, a memoir by Lucy's friend Ann Patchett (*Truth and Beauty*) is also unwittingly misleading in its portrayal of disability. Neither the obituary, nor Patchett's contribution, considered the wider societal and cultural context of Grealy's disfigurement. Lucy did not become aware of her problem by looking in a mirror; it was the stares and hostility of others that manifested as a problem for her: 'I was suddenly appalled at the notion that I'd been walking around unaware of something that was apparent to everyone else. A profound sense of shame consumed me.' In addition, it was the treatment to normalise her rather than the cancer per se which disfigured her. Moreover, by superficially linking her death to her discomfort with her facial appearance, rather than considering a dependence on painkillers for serial surgeries, the component of her problems caused by medical treatment is ignored.

It is noteworthy that shame is not exclusive to those with obvious disabilities or deformities. It occurs with many forms of illness; in the words of Dr David Biro, societal attitudes mark patients as alien; 'for whatever reason we manage to concoct at a given time in history: the wrong sexual orientation, sinful behaviour, or repressive personalities'. Society defines disability, and culture gives it meaning, according to anthropologist Robert Murphy, in his social history of paralytic illness, *The Body Silent*. 'The disabled are not a breed apart . . . they represent humanity reduced to its bare essentials.' The awkwardness of others, the avoidances and 'even outright hostility so often manifested toward them by the non-disabled are not the natural products of their own physical deficits, but, rather, expressions of deficiencies of perspective and character of those who so behave'.

LONELINESS AND ALONENESS

'In the end you suffer alone,' observes Lorrie Moore's fictional mother as she frantically tries to cope with her sick child. 'I was in this alone' was the stark realisation of Lucy when considering her childhood experience with cancer. The ill and the disabled become society's marginal people. The banality of their suffering, which happens in the background, while the world looks away, is captured in W. H. Auden's famous poem 'Musée des Beaux Arts':

About suffering they were never wrong,
The Old Masters: how well they understood
Its human position; how it takes place
While someone else is eating or opening a window or just
    walking dully along.

Similarly, in John Betjeman's 'Devonshire Street W.1', alluded to earlier, 'the sun still shines' on a street busy with 'merciless, hurrying Londoners' outside the consulting room, where a man has been given a terminal diagnosis. Tolstoy is even more direct about how quickly the ill become marginalised in 'The Death of Ivan Ilyich'. When Ivan returns home from the doctor, and tries to tell his wife about it:

> his wife listened to him, but in the middle of the account his daughter came in with her hat on: she was going out with her mother. With an effort she sat down briefly to listen to this boring stuff, but she could not take it for long, and her mother did not hear him out in full . . . something terrible, new and so significant was happening inside Ivan Ilyich that never had he experienced anything more significant than this in his life. And he alone knew about it, while all those around him did not understand or did not want to understand and thought that everything on earth was carrying on as before. This was what tormented Ivan Ilyich more than anything.

For all its universality, illness is an intensely personal and lonely business. When John Donne, poet and Dean of St Paul's, was laid low in 1623 with relapsing fever, probably typhus, he wrote one of the great accounts of illness (*Devotions Upon Emergent Occasions,* published in 1624), in which he is tormented by his isolation as a patient: 'As sickness is the greatest misery, so the greatest misery of sickness is solitude. . . . Solitude is a torment which is not threatened in hell itself.' This thought led him to ponder the connectedness of human lives, and to his famous injunction 'No man is an island'.

Loneliness close to despair was infused in the words of Jonathan Swift as he faced the prospect of illness alone (*In Sickness*, 1714):

. . . no obliging, tender Friend
To help at my approaching End,
My Life is now a burden grown
To others, e'er it be my own.

Friends and loved ones are the predominant resources for coping with significant illness. Sadly, awkwardness and a feeling of inadequacy often keep friends and acquaintances away from the person who is ill.

The importance of staying connected with comrades was highlighted by Christopher Hitchens: 'My chief consolation in this year of living dyingly has been the presence of friends.' Connection and community among those who are ill or disabled was also highlighted by the Australian art critic and journalist Robert Hughes, while he was on an assignment in Lourdes. In the foothills of the Pyrenees, the French town of Lourdes is known to Catholics as the site where the Virgin Mary is thought to have appeared in the nineteenth century, and to which thousands of pilgrims flock annually in pursuit of miraculous cures. There, the sceptical Hughes encountered an Irishman with quadruple amputations who was on his ninth annual visit. In response to Hughes's delicate enquiry regarding the disabled man's expectations, a sharp look was returned, as if Hughes were mad: 'What sort of fool d'you take me for? . . . I come here because I like to be with my own class of people.'

Loneliness is an enduring whole-body affliction, not a state of being alone but a conscious feeling of social separation, as emphasised by historian Fay Bound Alberti in her *Biography of Loneliness*. The relationship between loneliness and illness is complex and variable. In *Anatomy of Illness*, Norman Cousins describes the psychology of illness as a 'conflict between the terror of loneliness and the desire to be left alone'.

Sick people spend a lot of time alone with their thoughts. Their loneliness has increased as doctors have become distanced, with less time to spend with patients, in the clinic, on the ward, and perhaps most importantly, in relation to home visits by family doctors. For Robert McCrum, 'the terrible isolation of stroke and its aftermath' meant time to brood: 'All you can do while you are lying there is to organise your thoughts and make the most of your time.' One of the paradoxes of illness, observes McCrum, is 'the more everything is reported, analysed, expounded . . . in newspaper columns . . . and the more people feel able to express whatever they think, the more deafening the general silence that hangs over illness and ill-health'.

DISBELIEF AND DISMISSAL

The most unfair burden of chronic illness is the concern that, sooner or later, others might suspect that the illness is not real. Doubt arises if illness occurs without signs of disease, and patients feel the need to convince others as well as themselves of the reality of their illness, particularly when no cause is apparent. There is a lot wrong with medical labels, as discussed earlier, but this is one situation where a correct diagnostic label can help a patient cope with their illness.

The compulsion to play the sick-role compounds the illness. For example, the Nobel laureate Sir Peter Medawar believed that Charles Darwin was 'genuinely ill', although his multitude of complaints were unexplained,[9] and 'having nothing to show for it – surely a great embarrassment to a man whose whole intellectual life was a marshalling and assay of hard evidence'. According to Medawar, Darwin may have been like many patients suspected of hypochondria who have to 'pretend to be iller than they really are and may then get taken in by their own deception'. As succinctly stated by Nortin Hadler in a 1996 article in the medical journal *Spine*, 'if you have to prove you are ill, you can't get well'.

In an essay addressing the inadequacy of medical words to describe pain, Sinéad Gleeson emphasises 'unlistened to pain'. Declarations of pain, she says, are often met with doubt. 'I have been condescended to by enough consultants to know when I'm not believed.' The problem may be worse for women, for minority groups, and particularly for those with disorders which are controversial or poorly understood. Porochista Khakpour's 2018 memoir of chronic illness, *Sick*, explores the realities of living with undiagnosed chronic disease:

> the deal with so many chronic illnesses is that most people won't want to believe you. They will tell you that you look great, that it might be in your head only, that it is likely stress, that everything will be okay.

After years of feeling sick, and the 'hostile world of hospital rooms and doctors' offices', and 'the anger of being misunderstood', 'that feeling of not being taken seriously by those who had your life in their hands', Khakpour was diagnosed with chronic late-stage Lyme disease. Lyme disease is caused by a bacterial infection (with Lyme *Borrelia,* which include *Borrelia burgdorferi, Borrelia garinii* and others) transmitted to humans by tick-bites. Although the symptoms and signs, diagnosis and treatment of active Lyme disease are well described, false-positive diagnoses are common, and the question of chronic post-treatment Lyme disease is controversial. Khakpour writes: 'It's thought of as the disease of hypochondriacs and alarmists and rich people who have the money and time to go chasing obscure diagnoses. For years I'd become used to dealing with all sorts of skeptics whether in person or online, but it never stopped being frustrating.'

While conceding the scarcity of good data, Khakpour also contends that women suffer the most from Lyme, and tend to progress to late stages of the illness because doctors often treat them as psychiatric cases first. 'Women simply aren't allowed to be physically sick until they are mentally sick too.' Gender bias and sexism throughout medicine and the healthcare system have been well documented by several authors, most notably by journalist Maya Dusenbery, whose book *Doing Harm* is a revealing account of hidden and overt gender discrimination. Women find it more difficult than men to have their symptoms taken seriously; they wait longer than men for diagnostic tests, and for treatment in emergency rooms. This discrimination is particularly evident for women suffering with poorly understood conditions where illness is predominant without objective signs of disease.

GAIN

'Do not curse your fate; count your possibilities' is the advice given by Arthur Frank in his famous book of reflections on illness, *At the Will of the Body*. His examples of opportunities for gain – 'closer relationships, more poignant appreciations and clarified values' – may seem too abstract for those in the first throes of crisis. Acute sufferers with illness and disability have no need of patronising platitudes. However, over time many survivors with chronic illness come to appreciate that for all that they have lost through illness, there are possibilities for gain. Philosopher Havi Carel looks at chronic illness through the eyes of one afflicted with a serious progressive respiratory illness, and argues that well-being is achievable, and can co-exist with illness. Emily Dickinson alludes to the co-existence of loss and gain in her poem 'My first well Day – since many ill':

> My loss, by sickness – Was it Loss?
> Or that Ethereal Gain
> One earns by measuring the Grave –
> Then – measuring the Sun –

Attitudes to the notion of gain from illness have changed with improved understanding of illness. Clinicians once viewed gain from illness in a negative light because it linked the patient with blame. The term *secondary gain* refers to a conscious use of illness to derive benefit, social, occupational or otherwise, from others. In truth, the usefulness of the term has been challenged as it stereotypes many patients and is often confused with malingering, attention-seeking, compensation-seeking or medico-legal motivations. Such negative connotations diminish the majority of people, who need to be encouraged to explore whatever possibilities, opportunities or gains that illness may bring.

As we have seen, Barbara Ehrenreich has no truck with the concept of gain with illness. She is dubious of declarations, made with the benefit of hindsight, that illness has brought some form of gain for a patient, particularly a patient with cancer. She is distrustful of what she calls 'testimonies to the redemptive powers of the disease' and is rightfully distrusting of vacuous statements like that of the infamous bike-racer Lance Armstrong after his treatment for testicular cancer: 'Cancer was the best thing that ever happened to me.' She is angered by the effect of such sugar-coated language, which transforms cancer into a rite of passage rather than a tragedy, and which diminishes or denies the devastation inflicted by cancer on many patients.

In some instances, illness may be unconsciously influenced by what may be perceived as a form of gain. For example, Theodore Roosevelt, the twenty-sixth president of the United States (1901 to 1909), suffered from severe childhood asthma, the intermittent episodes of which gave him the opportunity to spend valued time with his father. This was shown many years after Roosevelt's death in a painstaking analysis of medical records by historian David McCullough, who emphasised that while Roosevelt's pattern of asthmatic attacks was influenced by apparent gain, the suffering was in no way lessened as a result.

In contrast, most patients have sufficient insight to openly acknowledge the few consoling gains they can mine from their illness. For example, artists, philosophers and scientists have transformed the solitude of illness into creative activity. Charles Darwin was beset with chronic illness but conceded that his symptoms saved him from the distractions of society.

Contemporary examples of unanticipated gain from illness or disability enrich our understanding of what it means to suffer and live with disadvantage. The Pulitzer Prize-winning poet Philip Schultz attributed his deep appreciation of language and music to dyslexia, which had remained undiagnosed until his son was diagnosed with the same condition. Out of shame, embarrassment and frustration when it came to enunciating words, he had found ways of manipulating and circumnavigating sounds to produce great poetry. Words, which once failed him, ultimately saved him: 'the very things I couldn't do have helped provide me with a profession and a means of knowing myself'. While speech is acquired subconsciously, reading must be learned consciously; Schultz recalls pretending to read, and would imagine the words before he could read them. He now uses this method to teach others who have the same problem.

Numerous other examples attest to the unanticipated gain that may arise with illness.[10] Entrepreneur and business tycoon Richard Branson traces much of his success with customer communication to his dyslexia, and Irish journalist Fintan O'Toole attributes his vocabulary and appreciation of the written word to a childhood stammer. Likewise, the life of Melody Gardot was transformed in her late teens from fashion student to accomplished musician and singer-songwriter. When she sustained serious injuries to her head, limbs and pelvis, she was left with significant disability, including a speech deficit. Music therapy to help 'reconnect neural pathways' in her brain did not eliminate her disabilities, but it did facilitate an innate ability that was to mature into the composition of original music – and, ultimately, international success.

In the end, illness transforms us. It inflicts a series of losses, but it also presents possibilities, which occasionally may be converted to gain.

TRUST

Patients do not have to like their carers, but they do need to trust them. 'The central question to be asked about hospitals – or about doctors for that matter – is whether they inspire the patient with confidence that he or she is in the right place; whether they enable [one] to have trust.' These were the words of Norman Cousins in his *Anatomy of an Illness*. In the forty years since the publication of that story, trust in doctors and tolerance of poor health services has declined. Some of this is warranted. A degree of scepticism is appropriate, but distrustful patients are disadvantaged: they are less likely to take prescribed medications or to adhere to medical advice, and may even adopt unhealthy habits. When trust is lost, anger takes its place.

'What I resented most about Dr Singer was that he made a practice of lying to me.' These are the words of Lucy Grealy, from her memoir of childhood cancer. Years went by before the word *cancer* was explicitly used – 'I thought I had a Ewing's sarcoma' – and as a child, she had not been told it was an aggressive form of cancer: 'Not one person ever said the word cancer to me, at least not in a way that registered as pertaining to me.' Later, she felt that she and the doctors were speaking 'two different languages'. After a disappointing operation, when doctors told her how well her face looked, she was devastated, and felt silly for having any expectations or hopes at all. Her reversed image in a mirror 'was the true image, the way other people saw me'.

Similarly, in Tolstoy's 'The Death of Ivan Ilyich', Ivan cannot trust those around him to acknowledge the truth of his decline with illness. Even with the doctor, 'it turned out that what the doctor had said to him was not what had been done. Either he had forgotten, or he had lied, or he was hiding something from him.'

A patient's trust in a doctor may be resolved into three critical questions, according to healthcare policy expert Dr Dhruv Khullar. The first relates to competence: 'Do you know what you are doing?' Second is transparency: 'Will you tell me?' The third relates to conflicts of interest: 'Are you doing it to help me or you?'

Rebuilding trust among patients, their doctors and their healthcare teams was the focus of the American Board of Internal Medicine Foundation at its annual retreat in 2018. An extensive list of proposed actions and strategies emerged.[11] However, most patients would probably summarise requirements in one or two words: honesty, truthfulness. This applies not only to individual practitioners but also to leaders of healthcare systems and those responsible for healthcare policy.

Trust in a doctor is no longer blind, nor can it be assumed. It takes time to foster. Diminishing time spent by doctors with their patients seems to be an obvious cause of loss of trust. Trust is also undermined by medical scandals, marketplace medicine, blatant advertising, triumphalist slogans and the advent of league tables of hospital performance, the distancing effect of the electronic health record, and specialisation, leading to multiple doctors being assigned to a single patient. Of course, trust is highly dependent upon expectations. Doctors should ask their patients: 'What is your goal for your healthcare, and how can I help you achieve it?' Commonly, a patient's expectation or goal differs from that of the doctor; remarkably, it may be far more modest than anticipated, and demand less intervention than expected. For their part, doctors earn the trust they deserve with time and honesty about the limits of medicine and its uncertainties. Transparency can be facilitated by sharing the computer screen and dictating letters to referring doctors in the presence of the patient. In the end, trust must be mutual, and is built over time, but it can be undermined quickly. Throwaway comments, little white lies (which are never *little* in medicine), lapses in confidentiality, or criticism of other doctors actually undermine patients' confidence in the entire profession.

Most people say that they trust their own doctor but frequently offer that they distrust the system, the institutions of medicine, including the hospitals, the politicians, and the media. Some of this loss of trust is due to obfuscation and other abuses of language – which are discussed later, in Chapter 12.

HUMOUR

Seemingly misplaced among the illness-words, humour features at some stage in many illness-stories. For some, it lightens the burden of illness; for others, humour offsets the awkwardness of friends who do not know what to say. Stand-up comics have used their own illness or disablement to make people laugh, and artists and writers have drawn on the comic absurdities of illness. The works of James Joyce abound with medical playfulness: 'he was shocking poor in his health, he said, with the shingles falling off him' (*Finnegans Wake,* 39.26).

Curiously, many patients seek relief from the boredom of illness and its treatment. 'Cancer is borin',' says the likeable Jimmy Rabbit, one of Roddy Doyle's characters in *The Guts*. Jimmy resorts to bar-room wit while drinking pints in the local pub, as he tells his father that he will be having surgery for colon cancer.

'They'll take out 80 percent of your . . . bowels?' asks Jimmy's father.

Somewhat assured that Jimmy will be able to function normally after the surgery, the father continues: 'With what's left?'

'Yeah,' replies Jimmy.

'The 20 percent,' persists the father, to which Jimmy retorts: 'Fair play. You were always good at the subtraction.'

Humour and irony are also used by people with physical disablement. In a memorable scene from the film *The King's Speech*, the royal family have assembled to view a Pathé newsreel of the Coronation, which is followed by a segment in which Adolf Hitler is shown mesmerising an audience, shouting and gesticulating with his mad eloquence: 'What's he saying, Papa?' says his older daughter, Elizabeth – to which the reluctant new King, who has been terrified of public speaking because of his stammer, replies: 'I don't know, but he seems to be saying it rather well.'

Even patients with major illness, including mental impairment, can laugh at their predicament. My favourite is the following conversation overheard from two elderly ladies with advanced Alzheimer's dementia, as they held on to each other, gingerly exiting a church pew after a religious service. Each was under close vigilance by their carers, because of repeated injuries from falls due to their frailty.

'Now Rose, you go first and I will follow,' said Mary.

'I will yeah . . . so that when I fall, you'll have a soft landing!'

Humour is, of course, a serious business. It is the exclusive prerogative of the patient, not the carer. In other words, the patient takes the lead, and only if invited should the carer join the banter. Seldom, if ever, should carers risk adding to the suffering by causing offence with an ill-timed witticism.

4

Waiting, Uncertainty and Time

WAITING[1]

'Nothing happens. Nobody comes, nobody goes. It's awful.'
—*Waiting for Godot,* Samuel Beckett

Waiting. It is an inescapable part of the human condition, perhaps; but it is also a big part of the experience of illness. Being ill is being patient. Why use such a word otherwise! 'Nobody, not even a lover, waits as intensely as a critically ill patient,' according to Anatole Broyard, in his unsentimental commentary on his own experience with prostatic cancer. Patients wait for results, wait for good or bad news, and in many health services, wait to see the doctor, and a specialist, and then another specialist. All patients wait for an outcome. Uncertainty. 'I don't know how this story will end': a bold declaration by a celebrity after public disclosure of her recovery from treatment for breast cancer.[2]

Everybody waits. In the 1991 motion picture *The Doctor*, a skilled and once insensitive surgeon reforms after he develops laryngeal cancer and encounters the bureaucratic inefficiencies of healthcare, which will be familiar to many patients: the errors, the endless forms to be filled in, and the waiting. Joining the press of human bodies in the waiting area, he expresses his frustration to neighbouring patients: I am a doctor' – to which a young woman suffering with a brain tumour replies: 'Not when you're sitting here.' Even the privileged and the celebrities wait at some phase of their illnesses. As Robert McCrum puts it: 'We are all, in some sense, in the doctor's waiting room.'

Medical waiting rooms differ from other waiting areas. More than a temporary halting site to pass through on the way to another destination, the medical waiting room completes the transformation of a person to a patient. In her essay on the medical waiting room, Laura Tanner refers to 'this atypical public space', which steals some of a patient's sense of control, poise and dignity. The configuration of most medical waiting rooms, regardless of décor, she writes, disallows any attempt to establish 'personal territory through the kind of purposeful posture and motion that occur so easily even in crowded locker rooms or transit waiting areas'. The medical waiting room renders public the illness – which is actually a private, personal condition. The acute self-awareness of the patient who is waiting, is heightened by anticipation of clinical scrutiny of one's body.

In her introduction to *The Poetry Cure*, Julia Darling comments on the disempowerment and helplessness experienced by patients while they are waiting in the surreal environment of a hospital. She restored her own sense of control by writing poems, many of which were begun in the waiting room:

> Acute ears listen for
> the call of our names . . .
> Our names, those dear consonants
> and syllables, that welcomed us
> when we began,
> before we learnt to wait . . . .

Elsewhere, a physician reflects in verse on the bonds securing a family in a waiting room against the 'flood of words and looks'.[3] For some, the waiting room is laden with suffering, a vivid separation of the ill from the well – but mainly a place where the poor go.[4] The medical waiting room has been assigned a persona unto itself by the English poet Ursula A. Fanthorpe:

> I am the room that understands waiting,
> With my box of elderly toys, my dog-eared *Women's Owns*,
> Permanent as repeat prescriptions, unanswerable as ageing,
> Heartening as the people who walk out smiling, weary
> As doctors and nurses working on and on.'

Another poet, Elizabeth Bishop, relives a childhood experience when she accompanied her aunt to a dental appointment. While in the waiting room, she had a dawning awareness of her own identity, becoming a little frightened of the gravity of her own existence in a world of grown-ups. As an adult, the poet recalls the episode, and the elements of the waiting room which contributed to a loss of some of her childhood innocence.

Artists have long been intrigued by stories of illness, and have expressed the emotions and context of illness in many forms. There are stories on the faces of patients in waiting rooms. L. S. Lowry captured these in his portrayal of *A Doctor's Waiting Room* (c. 1920) and *Ancoats Hospital Outpatients Hall* (1952), where lines of patients are arranged on benches like a mechanised conveyor leading to the doctor. These images are records of a bygone time, but the scenes presented by Lowry are as familiar and germane today as they were when they were created more than half a century ago.[5]

For some, the waiting experience is akin to that of a social gathering; for many, it is a solitary experience; and for a few, the anticipation of bad news is written on their faces. Doctors who are observant of patients waiting will recognise the stories on the faces immediately. Lowry's image is almost identical to my memory of the hospital where I trained; other than the décor, it looks much like where I now work. Indeed, a contemporary description of the outpatient department in an otherwise modern hospital is reminiscent of Lowry's scenes: 'The place is a maelstrom of patients, relatives, doctors, nurses, secretaries, porters, ambulance staff, students and the occasional dog.' [6] Curiously, it is a place where 'examples of senior management species are rarely encountered' – except when accompanying occasional 'political dignitaries, in anticipation of whose coming, the place has been sanitised and cleansed of all but a few token patients.'

While the experience of illness is individual and personal, the occurrence and facts of illness are universal; so it is with medical waiting rooms. An untitled photograph by Paul Seawright (c. 2006) of a woman and child waiting in a dishevelled clinic in sub-Saharan Africa addresses the difficulties of access to adequate healthcare in many parts of the world, while at the same time conveying the apprehension and boredom of waiting. A tired woman who appears to have a weight on her shoulders, sits patiently, surrounded by jaded public health posters and boxes, as her child, a toddler, still curious, looks toward the camera.

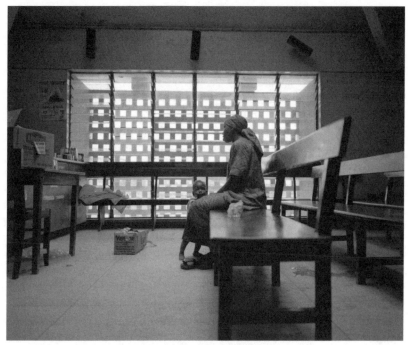

Untitled (Woman and Child), Paul Seawright
© *Paul Seawright. Reproduced by permission.*

'But outpatients are different', according to Ursula Farnthorpe, who experienced both sides of the divide, including a lengthy spell as an inpatient and, later, an outpatient department, where she worked as a clerk: 'They bring their kids with them, for one thing, and that creates a wrong atmosphere. They have shopping baskets and buses to catch. They cry, or knit' and 'they haven't yet learned/ How to be reverent.' This is a reminder to her overstretched healthcare colleagues that outpatients are real people with real lives to live.

In contrast, the poet likens hospital admission to an interview with St Peter at the gates of heaven, and addresses Peter ('I reckon, like me, you deal with the outpatients'), sharing with him the observation that the 'inpatients are easy' because they are under the control of the nurses and doctors and 'know what's what in the set-up'. Indeed, but inpatients wait in lonely isolation, after visiting hours, when a heightened awareness of body function may peak.

The design and organisation of hospitals is often suited more to institutional needs and acute care, with less attention to the needs of the chronically ill. This neglected aspect of the experience of illness is made more poignant by the striking images of the photographer Thomas Struth, which are separately selected for both the head and foot of each bed, to be viewed by the caregiver and the patient, respectively. Struth concentrates on subjects that might be 'missing': the images of local landscapes and flowers of intense colour, details of which are highlighted, reflecting the focal attention given to one part of the body during the experience of illness.

Waiting for death, the final struggle for a patient may also be a harrowing experience for vigilant loved ones, and for caregivers. To acknowledge and help assuage the guilt of those who silently wish for the death of a loved one or for another who suffers, John Humphrys and Sarah Jarvis, authors of a thoughtful work on the topic, used a provocative and telling title: *The Welcome Visitor*. Decay and death have intrigued artists through the ages.[7] In a monograph on waiting, the paintings by Ferdinand Hodler of the death of his mistress Valentine Godé-Dorel, are analysed.[8] In these famous images, the sufferer is alone. How should we behave in the face of another's suffering? The consensus appears to be: by saying 'here I am' – that is, by being there. Dying is what one must do by oneself, but no one should have to die alone.

Has waiting any value? For caregivers, waiting is not always attributable to delay and inefficiency; it may be intentional, a period to allow evolution of illness to clarify diagnosis or treatment. This is watchful or expectant waiting. For the patient, the interruption of time by illness is more than wasted time, it is experienced time. If 'too long a sacrifice/ can make a stone of the heart' for Yeats and 'hope deferred maketh the something sick' for Beckett, a temporary period of waiting provides respite from the non-essentials in life, an opportunity for redirecting attention to our values and relations with others. Like the experience of the imprisoned characters in Beckett's *Godot,* waiting while ill is always accompanied by an element of hope.

Uncertainty

I don't know how this story ends. Will the disease come back? Will the treatment work? How long will my response last? What is likely to happen? Patients usually have an intense desire to be rid of their fear of the unknown and the uncertain. Dr William Osler once famously declared that 'medicine is a science of uncertainty and an art of probability', to acknowledge that uncertainty is something that patients have in common with their doctors. Once was a time when a doctor's advice was presented with unquestioned God-like infallibility, seldom with any concession to doubt. Today, tolerating uncertainty has been described as the next medical revolution.

'You never know *for certain* about anything' says the brooding, self-questioning doctor in John Berger's classic 1967 study of a country doctor, *A Fortunate Man*. 'Most of the time you are right and you do *appear* to know, but every now and then the rules seem to get broken and then you realise how lucky you have been on the occasions when *you think you have known* and have been proved correct.' When doctors do not cope well with uncertainty, patients may suffer: too many tests, withholding of information, premature closure of decision-making process (thereby allowing hidden assumptions and unconscious biases to have more weight than they should, with associated increased risk of error).

The case for reducing clinical uncertainty in order to improve decision-making seems self-evident. Accurate prognostic information reduces unrealistic expectations and requests for expensive or ineffective treatments, while facilitating advance care planning and informed patient choice. However, the pursuit of absolute certainty is illusory. Uncertainty is a reality that needs to be acknowledged by patients and their care-providers. Moreover, some patients neither ask for nor wish to hear details of their prognosis. This is not denial; rather, it may reflect a *need* for uncertainty. Uncertainty has a value, in that it leaves open the possibility of hope.[9]

As counter-intuitive as it may seem to address uncertainty in terms of value, tolerance of uncertainty is more than a form of coping. It should be embraced as an opportunity for patients and their doctors to engage and reflect at a more meaningful level, and to escalate the patient-doctor interaction to one of partnership. In a time when access to information is no longer limiting, wisdom is a more important currency, and the role of a physician will increasingly become more akin to that of a counsellor supporting patients to manage risk and uncertainty as they navigate the complexities of the healthcare system. How can this be achieved?

As a patient, I would try to find a doctor who is curious about me, and about the unknown – and the uncertainty that my future presents. This would be a doctor who uses uncertainty to explore knowledge gaps, and one who acknowledges the difference between illness-uncertainty and disease-uncertainty. For all the uncertainty there may be with disease, the lived experience of that disease (illness) is vastly more uncertain and more complex. As a physician, I learned that confidence is not the same as certainty. Uncertainty can be communicated confidently without undermining credibility or perceived expertise, without igniting fear. 'I don't know' are some of the most important words in medicine; without them, honesty and trustworthiness in the doctor-patient relationship cannot survive. I have also learned the wisdom of words attributed to Voltaire: 'Doubt is not a pleasant condition, but certainty is an absurd one.'

TIME

> You can't see, touch, smell, or taste it, but we spend tens of billions on it every year. To many patients and their physicians, it is precious, may be the most precious of all medical resources. Yet we know only a little about how to use it efficiently or about the impact of using more or less of it. . . . It is, of course, time.
> —Dr Frank Davidoff, editor *Annals of Internal Medicine,* 1997

The greatest gift one can give the ill is one's time. Sick people experience time in ways that differ from the ways their carers do. Nowhere is the distinction between public or shared time, and lived or private time, more evident than during illness, when awareness of the quality and quantity of time becomes intense. The past is considered with fondness, regret or guilt, and the future becomes one of uncertainty and altered plans. Perception of the present is also transformed. Whereas the public perception of shared time is linear, the perception of time by those who are sick becomes cyclical, and akin to that of ancient humankind. Ancestral humans saw cyclical time in nature, with recurring sunrises and sunsets, the tides, the phases of the moon, and the seasons. Cyclical time is particularly important for the chronically sick, who live through relapses and remissions of illness. Small things become noticeable to the ill, and seemingly insignificant events in nature become important. Those with terminal illness wonder whether they will ever experience natural cycles and seasons again.

> Alice: 'How long is forever?'
> White Rabbit: 'Sometimes just one second.'

Although these familiar lines don't actually appear in the original *Alice*, they capture both the relativity of time and the reality that a life can pass in a split-second. Illness may strike in an instant, but then time slows down for the ill. Time becomes another element of the asymmetry of the patient-doctor relationship. As life slows down for the person in crisis, it continues apace for the other. It is the same with grief. Why can't the world stop? Why must life go on! Or to borrow from Auden: 'Stop all the clocks'. In extreme cases, time does seem to stop: consider Miss Havisham in Dickens' *Great Expectations,* and the Havisham-like experience of Queen Victoria after the death of her husband, Prince Albert.

Time becomes more meaningful than material things for those who are ill. 'How long will it take to see the doctor? How long do I have to wait for the test . . . for the operation . . . for the tablets to work . . . for the pain to go, for . . . for . . . for . . . ? How much time do I have left? I wish I had spent more time with . . . . I wasn't given enough time to explain.' For the ill, time passes like a snail, as the world spins, and people sail by.

'The velocity of the ill, however, is like that of the snail', wrote Emily Dickinson.[10] Likewise, for Elizabeth Tova Bailey, 'time continued to drag me along its path' when she was bedridden with illness. In her extraordinary and beautifully written book *The Sound of a Wild Snail Eating,* Bailey weaves an account of her illness with observations of a snail given to her by a visitor as a way of connecting with nature while she was bed-bound. 'We are all hostages of time,' she writes. 'My illness brought me such an abundance of time that time was nearly all I had. My friends had so little time that I often wished I could give them what time I could not use. It was perplexing how in losing health I had gained something so coveted but to so little purpose.' By the end of her book, Bailey, improved but still ill with chronic fatigue syndrome, had learned much from the snail. It had shown her a future with much that can be achieved while life goes on: 'Lots to do at whatever pace I can go. I must remember the snail.'

Time slows down when humans are thrown into a crisis, a frightening event, or a life-threatening illness. Scientists believe that this is not due to a sharpening of the perception of the passage of time but, rather, relates to the brain switching on a more enriched recording of memory for the event than normally operates in non-threatening situations. Regardless of how it occurs, the slowing of time is a consistent feature of illness-memoirs. Time and memory are tightly intertwined, and difficult to tease apart. The brain lays down less memory when events are familiar, and time then seems to pass more quickly. In contrast, the more detailed the memory, the more time seems to take longer. That's why time seems to speed up in old age and pass slowly in youth.

Distortions of time-perception are featured in several accounts of the experience of illness. In John Donne's classic meditation on his illness, time seemed to slow down and pass unnaturally:

> daies and nights, so long, as that Nature herself shall seeme to be perverted, and to have put the longest day, and the longest night, which should bee six moneths asunder, into one natural, unnaturall day.

Time-perception during illness is also one of the sub-themes of Thomas Mann's *The Magic Mountain*, in which the protagonist, Hans Castorp, visits an alpine sanatorium catering for patients with tuberculosis. Intending to stay three weeks, he ends up staying for seven years: 'I shall never cease to find it strange that the time seems to go so slowly in a new place . . . nothing whatever to do with reason, or with the ordinary ways of measuring time; it is purely a matter of feeling.' The narrator of the story continually struggles with the difficulty with time perception: 'Can one tell – that is to say, narrate – time, time itself, as such for its own sake? . . . For time is the medium of narration, as it is the medium of life. Both are inextricably bound up.' Illness turns patients inward, away from the world, and the external cues that sensitise us to the passage of time. A sense of time is unlike other senses, which are discrete non-overlapping ways of assessing our environment. A sense of time, however, integrates information from all other senses: 'For in yourself you have no sense-organ to help you judge of time or space.'

'What is the value of a moment?' This is the question posed repeatedly by John Berger in *A Fortunate Man*. The doctor, notes Berger, is preoccupied with time. 'The anguished are trapped in a moment,' he writes. 'Anguish has its own time-scale'; 'What separates the anguished person from the unanguished is a barrier of time'. Anguish relates to the sense of loss brought about by illness; adults with serious illness may become trapped in a moment that slows down to the time-scale of their childhood.

Night-time assumes a different significance for those who are ill. Pain and other symptoms are usually worse at night, when one is alone and there is reduced environmental stimulation. 'Nocturnal ordeal' is how Tony Judt described his suffering with motor neurone disease at night. 'Worst of all were the endless nights,' wrote Arnold Relman in his account of his utter helplessness while recovering in hospital from a broken neck. While waiting through the night for the return of his wife, family, and rounds by teams of physicians, he 'slept very little and spent most of the time watching the minutes go by on the big wall clock in my room, waiting for daylight'.

Time is the defining feature of chronic illness, but time does not heal, as in Emily Dickinson's poem: 'Time never did assuage – An actual suffering strengthens . . . Time is a Test of Trouble – But not a Remedy'. Time, it is said, is Nature's way of ensuring that everything doesn't happen at once. But illness is often chaotic, and sometimes everything *does* happen at once. This is the problem with linear stories of illness and disability. Not every illness-story has a beginning, middle and end. Linear narratives attempt to put order on disorder, coherence where there is incoherence, and meaning where this is none. Chronic illness often has an indeterminate beginning, a variable course and an uncertain future. Moreover, chronic illness may veer from prolonged periods of control to unpredictable cycles of relapse, which cannot be captured by linear narratives. It is not something to be triumphed over nor defeated by.

The ancient Greeks had two words for time, to distinguish quality and the value of a moment (*kairos*) from quantity (*chronos*). This distinction has renewed importance for patients with chronic cyclical diseases.

5

⊰⊰⊰

It's the Way You Say It

'It is not what you say that matters but the manner in which you say it;
there lies the secret of the ages.'

—William Carlos Williams (1883-1963)[1]

*Epiphanies – Chitchat – Loose Talk – Questions – Real-speak – Framing
the Question – Framing Risk – Leading Questions – Interruptions –
Mending Mindsets – Coaching Not Coaxing – Plain Language and Clean
Language – No Claptrap – Social Media Medicine*

Just words, but important words: get them right, and they become
powerful. This message has been demonstrated many times in
different formats, but a YouTube video made in Glasgow a decade ago
is particularly compelling.[2] It shows a blind man begging in public with
a sign: 'I'm blind please help.' Passers-by drop an odd coin, but their
response changes when a young woman pauses and changes the words
on the blind man's sign to read: 'It's a beautiful day and I can't see
it.' The new words have power because they link fact with emotion.
Ordinary and abstract are transformed into something personal.

The importance of the choice of words is played out every day in
every discussion between a patient and a doctor. Developing a keen ear
for the subtleties of how patients express their problems is rewarding
not only as a skill in itself but also as one of the pleasures of clinical
medicine. Every clinician can cite remarkable epiphanies expressed
in the words of patients; some favourites from my clinical time are
included in the next section.

Epiphanies

Most of what I've learned about chronic illness, I've learned from patients.
Persuading patients that their best option for controlling disease is
adherence to recommended treatments is my usual role. On the other
hand, poignant words used by patients are a continual reminder that only

the patient knows how the treatment of disease impacts the lived experience of disease. The words of three patients are particularly memorable.

John was a quiet young man with inflammatory bowel disease who was referred to me for an expert opinion on whether he should opt for surgical removal of his colon with the creation of a permanent stoma (an opening on the abdomen connected to the intestine, allowing waste to be diverted to a bag outside the body).[3] I was the last in a long series of specialists who had been consulted – all of whom had recommended the surgery. There was no doubt about the severity of John's disease, judging from his medical records. Nor did he lack information: he had already met a stoma therapist and spoken with patients who had undergone the same type of surgery. Moreover, two accompanying sisters were intent on making me aware that they were sure that surgery was long overdue. John's answers to my questions were direct, and confirmed his suffering. I had no reason to disagree with the previous advice. I asked what his thoughts were on the matter. His response changed everything. Nervously, in a halting voice, John said: 'I know that if I have the surgery it would be easier . . . easier for the doctors and the nurses . . . but it wouldn't be easier for me.'

Immediately we switched the discussion from surgery toward the optimal use of drug treatments, with attention to detail. My revised plan was to help John live with his condition until he could cope with the prospect of surgery, but over time, the necessity for surgery receded. We were able to manage the condition effectively by non-surgical means thereafter.

The words of another patient were no less remarkable in how they profoundly changed the way in which she was treated. This was Rose, a middle-aged woman with no specific complaints, and no active disease. But all was not well: she had been successfully treated with surgery for Crohn's disease of the small intestine many years earlier, and had a stoma. Her husband was supportive, downplayed the stoma, and offered that it never affected the couple's intimacy. She wasn't seeking a reversal of the stoma, but when asked directly how it affected her, she thought for a moment, and then said: 'I feel like I *am* the stoma. I feel like a big stoma.' Hearing herself say these words, this uncomplaining woman realised that she was living with profound distortions of body-image and her sense of self. This opened the way for a discussion balancing the theoretical risk of a relapse of Crohn's disease against the psychological benefit of a surgical take-down of the stoma, with restoration of bowel continuity. Neither she nor I had any doubt that her mental health and well-being was worth the risk.

Then there was David, the pleasant young man who was a regular attender at the inflammatory bowel disease clinic. He seemed to be a loner, with no family support, and had previously been diagnosed with Crohn's disease by another clinician. David's symptoms seemed disproportionate to any physical findings, and there was no objective evidence for active Crohn's disease. On review of his records, the evidence for the original diagnosis seemed weak. For most people, Crohn's disease, even when quiescent, is a substantial burden, with economic implications relating to employment and medical insurance. Thinking that I might be able to relieve this man of an unnecessary burden and label, his words were strikingly insightful: 'Oh doctor, you're not going to take my Crohn's disease away, are you? It's all that I have.'

CHITCHAT

Clinical conversations occasionally turn at a critical moment, a point when a patient divulges a painful truth, which has hitherto lain hidden. It takes time for patients to have trust. Trust doesn't come easily, and may never be given up to doctors who are in a hurry. It is not surprising that stories told by physicians about these moments of connection have in common the time taken to express curiosity in the patient's story, which only unfolds during what may seem like small talk. Chitchat takes time, but it is not wasted time. In a timeless essay entitled 'Communion' by Dr Richard Weinberg, a young lady presents with abnormal bowel movements but seems disproportionately distressed. Several consultations are required before she is willing to elaborate on an event in her background that is contributing to her symptoms, and then only when Weinberg and she discover in conversation that they have a shared passion for baking.

Sometimes, the diagnostic epiphany is neither painful nor known to the patient. I recall such a moment after seeing a retired man with perplexing episodes of severe hepatitis (liver inflammation). After consulting several doctors, he arrived at my office and announced what no doctor likes to hear: 'Doctor, you're my last resort.' He was polite, had little confidence that I might be of any help, and was firm in his resolve not to have any more tests: 'I've already had the Rolls-Royce of investigations several times,' he declared. Apparently, I wasn't the first to notice the obvious in his voluminous records: the acute abnormalities in his liver tests were severe but episodic, and were followed by a full, albeit temporary, return to normal. My questions regarding the usual culprits for liver damage were tediously familiar to him. He didn't drink too much alcohol, and no, 'Before you ask, I've never consumed dodgy mushrooms, herbs or drugs.' I told him that I had no idea what was wrong with him. I agreed not to request another liver biopsy or more tests. Then he relaxed and we chatted about life after retirement. Retirement, he said, was emancipation. If only he could be free of his hepatitis, he would have more time to pursue his only passion: shooting game-birds during the season. As a city-slicker, I knew nothing about game-birds, but was curious about his guns. This led to a series of questions which revealed that 'the season' correlated with his episodes of 'hepatitis'. Then, an avalanche of information unfolded, and established that the material he used to clean his guns contained carbon tetrachloride, one of the most potent of liver toxins, consumed by inadvertent inhalation. No tests needed. Case closed thanks to curious chitchat.

Loose Talk

In contrast to chitchat, which is interactive and constructive, loose talk is overheard and idle, and undermines a patient's confidence. Everyone involved in the care of someone needs continual reminders that when a patient is present, he or she must be the centre of attention, and the distinction between crisis and routine must be respected. Too often this respect breaks down during procedures on unsedated patients, such as wound-dressing, plaster-applications, X-ray tests or endoscopies, when carers are distracted, or ignore the patient by discussing unrelated trivia. Patients in crisis don't need to hear about last night's party, karaoke, or pub quiz. Likewise, grumbling about working conditions, waiting lists, defective equipment, and slow retrieval of laboratory results, has a negative impact on patients' morale. More serious lapses of professionalism occur in corridors, cafeterias and elevators: hotspots where medical staff may inadvertently breach confidentiality by discussing 'cases'.

Questions

'Did you tell the doctor that?'
    'No.'
    'Why not?'
    'He didn't ask.'
    Who hasn't overheard or participated in such an exchange! I'm with the one being questioned. There is, of course, shared responsibility for the effectiveness of patient-doctor dialogue, but it falls to the physician to follow the patient's lead, not only to ask the right questions, but to ask them in the right way.

When I moved to Ireland after many years working in the United States and Canada, one of my new colleagues reminded me of the nuances of English as spoken in Ireland. Consider the question 'Will you take the tablets?' If a Corkman or woman says 'Yes', this single affirmative means that he or she will assuredly adhere to the treatment regimen. If, however, the response to the question is 'I will yeah', this double-affirmative is actually a negative, and means that the patient will not take the tablets. To complicate matters, some use a modified single affirmative 'I will in my ass [or other expletive]'; this, unlike the unmodified single affirmative, is a negative. To further complicate the matter, the Irish find it difficult to say no, and their expression of a negative is more colourful and varied than the affirmative.

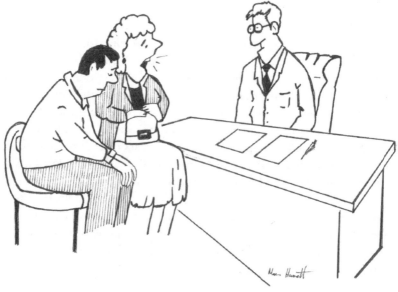

English as spoken in Cork (after Dr Gary Lee)

'He don't know, Doctor': the single negative.
'He don't know nothin', Doctor': the double negative.
'He don't know nothin' but feck all, Doctor': the triple negative.
'Ye don't know no one else who don't want nothin' done, do yeh, Doctor?': the poly-negative which sounds like an affirmative.[4]

I was to learn later that what a patient says, and how he or she responds to my questions, is influenced by what I say. Consider, for example, the question of tobacco-smoking and health. For some patients, such as those with Crohn's disease, any level of smoking may adversely affect their disease activity. Therefore, accuracy in history-taking on this point is particularly important.

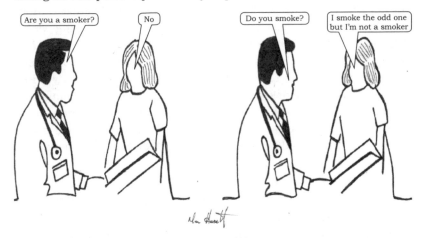

A simple change of language alters the response, because it invokes the link between the patient's self-regard and their behaviour. The effect of labelling the behaviour with a noun ('Are you a smoker?') rather than a verb ('Do you smoke?') changes the response. This is not only important in terms of framing a question but is also the first step to encouraging a change in behaviour and the adoption of a healthier lifestyle. Admitting to a harmful behaviour such as smoking is more acceptable to most patients than being labelled as a smoker. In other words, people's desire to shape their own identities can be harnessed to change behaviour. This rationale has been applied in reverse to motivate voter turnout in US elections. Invoking the self is the key strategy. For example, people are more inclined to vote in response to the question 'Are you a voter?' than if they are asked 'Are you going to vote?'[5] Thus, in the case of a desirable behaviour, the noun-label (voter) is acceptable, but in the case of undesirable behaviour, the noun-label (smoker) is less acceptable.

Real-speak

When Alice asked Humpty Dumpty whether he could make words mean different things, the hard-boiled Dumpty replied: 'They've a temper, some of them. Particularly verbs: they're the proudest. Adjectives you can do anything with, but not verbs.'

Politicians like to use sentences without verbs. This is because sentences without verbs make for good rhetorical soundbites without committing the speaker ('Better health for all', 'A kinder, gentler nation', 'Safer hospitals in the future'). Medicine is full of nouns and adjectives, but doctors should use verbs more, according to the linguist Dariusz Galasinski. This is because people tell their stories using verbs. Patients do not *have presentations with* pain, they *feel* pain. They *hurt* and they *bleed*, *cry* and *scream*. They *call on* doctors and *ask for* help. Similarly, people don't say 'There is love between us', they say 'I love you'. They should be asked how they feel, not what their feelings are. Doctors should also ask patients about *how* they understand what is happening, not *what* their understanding is. This is how real people speak, and that should be good enough for medical practitioners.

FRAMING THE QUESTION

Which would you prefer, a hamburger that is advertised as '80 percent lean beef' or one that is labelled '20 percent fat'? Either way, it's the same burger, but most people would opt for the former and reject the latter. Marketing analysts have exploited the persuasive effects of words that work and words that don't, for many decades. Curiously, the importance of word-choice has received insufficient attention in medicine and health, except perhaps when it is abused by defensive politicians and officialdom.

> When criticised for the poor quality of the health service, the politician responded by citing the patient experience survey. 'Over 80 percent of patients expressed satisfaction with their hospital experience,' he said, with a self-congratulatory smile. He didn't say that '20 percent were dissatisfied with their experience and about half of the patients did not respond to the questionnaire'. One in every five patients unhappy with their hospital experience is not a matter for self-congratulation.

Framing the statement in positive terms with a high number (80 percent) sounds better if you are defending the health service, but the same data when expressed as a percentage of dissatisfaction is indefensible.

FRAMING RISK

'Doctors don't take risks, patients do', according to the old adage. Sick people are often called upon to make vital decisions at times of crisis, when they are stressed and have impaired judgement. They depend on the accuracy of the explanation of risk and benefit provided by carers. Explaining risk is difficult, and must be tailored to the needs and capacity of the patient to understand it. Compounding this, is the high level of uncertainty in all medical situations. Moreover, patients will often make a decision based on emotions rather than facts. The kindness, competence and trustworthiness of the doctor are critical.

Descriptive words such as *low* and *high* risk may mean different things to different people. Words should be supported with numbers and images, but there are some ground-rules which have been recommended by risk communication experts. All patients need to be informed that there is no such thing as zero risk, and all therapeutic risk should be presented in the context of benefit over no treatment at all. In addition, absolute numbers are preferable to relative risks. For example, it is easy for a patient to misinterpret statements like 'The risk of cancer is increased by three times' if the actual risk is negligible. A baseline risk of 1 in 1000 increasing to 3 in 1000 is still a very small risk.

Statistics are indigestible for people in crisis. In Lorrie Moore's story of a child afflicted with a rare form of kidney cancer, the doctors tell the parents that 'the chances of this happening . . . to one kidney are one in fifteen thousand' and 'the chances on the second kidney are about one in eight'. 'One in eight,' says the Husband. 'Not bad. As long as it's not one in fifteen thousand.' This passage encapsulates a critical error when it comes to explaining risk, and the difficulty in understanding it. The odds of possible outcomes should always be presented with a consistent denominator: for example, 1 out of 15,000 and 1875 out of 15,000. With different denominators, many patients confuse which is the greater risk. Deception by denominators is frequently exploited as a marketing strategy. For example, if it is intended to give the impression of a low cost, a small scale is selected ($1 per day), whereas the same item seems far more expensive if a large scale is used ($365 per year).

Different ways of saying the same thing do not always produce the same response. The same is true with numbers, and the format in which they are presented. Classic experiments by the Nobel laureate Daniel Kahneman and the late Amos Tversky, showed how numerical framing has a modifying influence on people's judgements and decisions, as shown in the following example:

> *If 600 people are expected to die in an outbreak of a rare disease, which of the two proposed strategies to combat the disease will you adopt?*
> *With Strategy A, 200 people will be saved.*
> *With Strategy B, there is a 1/3 chance that 600 people will be saved and a 2/3 chance that no one will be saved.*

Most people are risk-averse and go for the certainty of strategy A, foregoing the risk of not saving anyone. However, the results are different when the problem is re-framed as follows:

> *With Strategy C, 400 people will die.*
> *With Strategy D, there is a 1/3 chance that nobody will die and a 2/3 chance that 600 will die.*

Now, most people opt for Strategy D because they are averse to the certainty of loss and are willing to take a big risk to avoid it. Of course, the outcomes of Strategy A and Strategy C are the same (200/600 saved = 400/600 lost) but the choice was influenced by the way in which the options were framed.

Susceptibility to the vagaries of numerical framing is not limited to novices; experts are similarly affected, and framing bias affects both doctors and patients. In a remarkable study published in the *New England Journal of Medicine*, McNeil, Tversky and colleagues assessed the preferences of patients and physicians for different forms of treatment for lung cancer. The way in which the information was presented had a striking influence on the results. Participants were asked whether they would opt for either surgery or radiation therapy if they were to develop lung cancer, and were provided with cumulative probabilities and life-expectancy data. For both patients and physicians, there was little difference in the proportions opting for either surgery or radiation if the expected results were expressed in terms of mortality (probability of dying), whereas surgery tended to be the preferred option if the same data were presented in terms of probability of living (survival framing).[6]

Simple tools have been devised by John Paling and others to help patients and doctors assess medical risks. Visual aids are especially useful for patients with poor numeracy or literacy skills, and are an advisable supplement to any discussion of risk. For example, for a medical risk with a probability of greater than one in one thousand, a picture of a thousand miniature human images can be used, the proportion of which is encircled or highlighted to represent the actual probability or risk per thousand subjects. An advantage of this pictorial format is that it can simultaneously show actual numbers unambiguously for the estimates of positive outcomes and negative outcomes.

LEADING QUESTIONS

A successful patient-doctor interview should be two-directional, with meaningful pauses and attentive listening on both sides. As the clinician gathers information about the patient's condition (history-taking), the patient is knowingly or unknowingly assessing the clinician, seeking reassurance of being in competent hands. The style of questioning has a profound influence on the accuracy of the information gathered, and on the patient's evaluation of the physician. Doctors are taught to ask unbiased, open-ended questions. Patients quickly recognise that repetitive use of leading questions ('You don't smoke, do you?' or 'You didn't vomit, did you?') can distract or re-direct the conversation away from the main problem. Leading questions tend to bias the questioner toward their initial impressions (anchoring bias) and generate information to support the doctor's prior and perhaps mistaken belief (confirmation bias). These pitfalls are well known but all rules are meant to be broken – otherwise the sun would still be orbiting the earth!

Rarely, because of the limitations of illness-language, a leading question becomes appropriate. This arises in the case of the common condition irritable bowel syndrome, the diagnosis of which relies exclusively on symptoms. If given time, most patients volunteer without prompting an accurate description of symptoms compatible with the diagnosis, but some bowel disturbances may go unidentified because they defy description in ordinary terms. An example is the sense of incomplete evacuation after an intended bowel-movement, to a degree that the patient finds it difficult to leave the toilet-bowel. This is quite characteristic of irritable bowel syndrome; it is an important diagnostic point but often requires a prompt in the form of a leading question from the clinician. As we will see in Chapter 9, failure to clarify this point has led to misclassification of patients with irritable bowel syndrome – with disastrous complications when they were treated with an experimental drug.

INTERRUPTIONS

The medical interview is a conversation not an interrogation. Like most business meetings, the medical interview is more efficient if the agenda is set at the outset. Ideally, the patient should be asked to outline the agenda (with a list of concerns or problems), and then should be invited to elaborate, with the reasonable expectation of having sufficient time without interruption. In two famous studies of audiotaped medical interviews fifteen years apart, it was found that in over two-thirds of cases, doctors interrupted their patients within about twenty seconds.[7] Early interruptions are particularly problematic, because, once interrupted, patients tend not to raise additional concerns – some of which may be more important than the first item they raise, and which remain 'hidden'.

Of course, not all interruptions are intrusive; some may be cooperative. Respectful redirection of the patient may be needed to maintain focus. Details often need clarification to pursue a diagnosis, and to ensure common understanding of what has been said. Some interruptions may show encouragement by offering a cue or missing word, and build rapport. Doctors need to distinguish facts in the medical history from interpretations and inferences. Equally, doctors need to establish whether the patient is using his or her own words, or unwittingly repeating words and interpretations picked up from earlier consultations. Context and common sense are important, but patients are entitled to more than twenty seconds of silence from their doctor while they recount their illness-story.

MENDING MINDSETS

The outcome of all doctor-patient encounters is influenced by mindsets, which include the beliefs and expectations of both the doctor and the patient, and the appropriateness of each of these to the situation. An expectation of a healing, in contrast to despair and disbelief, is more likely to yield a favourable outcome. In this respect, the doctor's language is a key modifier of expectations. For example, controlled studies have shown that when drug prescriptions are accompanied with positive information from the doctor, outcomes are measurably better.

Modifying mindsets involves no deception, and in that respect differs from placebos (dummy tablets or sham treatments), which are discussed in Chapter 7. Doctors and carers act out a role of modifying patients' mindsets on a daily basis. Their choice of words is important for patients' outcomes, but the time and effort spent in this role is poorly appreciated by health-service bureaucracies.

Likewise, time and careful language are needed to offset adverse pre-conceptions and negative mindsets. For example, a despairing attitude toward chronic disease is particularly common in adolescents: 'I've tried everything and nothing works' or 'It's hopeless, I'm just a bad patient' or 'My mother had the same thing. It's in my genes.' Pessimism can be offset by switching the language from cure to control, and by explaining that lifestyle can trump genes, and by using stories of patients who beat the odds and gained control over their condition. Positive, confident statements are needed to re-shape the mindset: 'Don't deny the diagnosis, defy the verdict', 'The prognosis is not determined by statistics', 'Don't let the disease control you, you control the disease' and 'We will be there to help you take control.' Some doctors are more convincing than others, and some patients are less responsive than others, but one thing is certain: this kind of coaching is a central, not a supplementary, element of caring for chronic disease.

COACHING NOT COAXING

Doctors often assume that communicating advice and information about health behaviours is a sufficient investment of effort on behalf of their patients. This may work for a minority of patients, but it is usually insufficient, even when delivered with exactitude and clarity. Most patients listen politely, and many try to heed advice in good faith, but when this advice is delivered in a one-way, doctor-to-patient consultation, good intentions fade and many patients will eventually resist. As with any form of learning, didactic one-way receipt of information is less effective than active participation and engagement by the learner with the teacher: the same is true for health information. Simply telling people the facts may have a short-term effect, but is less likely to have a sustained impact, unless it achieves true commitment. Managing emotions is more important than facts and logic. In other words, when persuading patients to change, it is not enough to provide them with winning facts; one must win them over. Nurses are often better in this context than doctors: they tend to be less didactic, to listen better; they may also be regarded as more approachable by patients.

Doctors *and* nurses overestimate how much patients understand or recall what they have been told. Moreover, in some instances, only about half of patients adhere to prescribed medications. The adherence rates are much worse when it comes to advice regarding lifestyle and healthcare behaviour.

A more effective way to help patients change their behaviour involves two-way conversation among equals, in which the wisdom and resourcefulness of the patient is acknowledged and explored. With dialogue (not monologue), it is accepted that the outcome is uncertain, but the solution for the patient is likely to be found within the patient's own resourcefulness. This is the essence of coaching. Coaching is facilitating the patient's active participation in managing their own health. The doctor is the facilitator, helping to empower the patient by exploring possibilities.

A growing body of information suggests that patients who receive coaching are more likely to change and become motivated to adopt healthful behaviours. Likewise, when the clinician acts as coach, patients frequently report that the experience is more satisfying, less stressful, and more effective. The skills required for successful coaching are not difficult to learn, though becoming an outstanding coach may require many years of work/practice. Jenny Rogers, who is an executive coach, and Arti Maini, a clinician, have summarised the requirements succinctly in their book *Coaching for Health*: 'The mindset of the clinician who uses coaching is characterised by curiosity, neutrality and warmth.' Curiosity is needed to explore what the patient says and doesn't say; neutrality is about giving time, and attentive listening; and warmth is self-evident. The tactics are to put the patient in control; to guide self-care, adapted to the individualism of each patient; to prioritise goal-setting; and, of course, to emphasise precision of language.

Plain Language and Clean Language

Since the premise of coaching is that patients are themselves an important resource in healthcare, making best use of this resource requires doctor-patient consultations to be conducted through the medium of plain language. By substituting plain language for jargon and techno-speak, the asymmetric doctor-patient relationship may be re-balanced. There is a worldwide movement under way to promote plain language at all levels of society. Healthwise Incorporated, a non-profit company founded in the 1970s, provides patients and healthcare providers with information expressed in plain language, so that they can make better decisions. Most healthcare services pay some lip-service in support of plain language, but sadly, in many cases they continue with opaque circumlocution. In the late 1990s, the American vice president Al Gore famously said: 'Plain language is a civil right.' If so, it is a right that has been violated repeatedly. The language of deceit is never plain. But plain language is not a new concept. In Chaucer's *Canterbury Tales*, written in the fourteenth century, the Host exhorts the learned Clerke of Oxenford to speak plainly, without highfalutin' language, to the pilgrims so that they may understand him:

> Speketh so pleyn at this tyme, we yow preye,
> That we may understonde what ye seye.

The goal of plain language is to help the listener or reader make informed decisions. To achieve this, plain language rejects unnecessary jargon, but does not avoid essential complicated terms and concepts. Plain language is not a dumbing-down. Moreover, while plainness and precision may need to be balanced in the interest of clarity and usefulness, accuracy should never be compromised.

Related to plain language is the concept of clean language. This means that the patient's words are used to ensure that the clinician fully understands the emotional dimensions of the patient's experience of illness. The language is simple and positive, without casual or throwaway remarks, which are easily misconstrued and potentially hurtful, and often linger in patients' minds. Clean language is the currency of coaching. Its premise is that time spent on the language used by patients is a valuable investment for helping the patient make better decisions, and for both patient and physician to reach an improved understanding of the problems facing the patient. Clean language is not a tool of persuasion. Rather, it is a means for speaker and listener to achieve a more complete understanding of each other. In a clinical consultation, clean language requires attentive listening, and using the patient's own words and metaphors, not learned metaphors from the doctor. This helps the doctor to formulate questions to explore what the patient is thinking, to accurately state the problems, and to formulate potential solutions. The interviewer's language should contain as few assumptions as possible, and use only the patient's metaphors. The objective is to avoid the hindrance that language may pose, and to use language that helps the patient to reach a clearer understanding of themselves and to achieve a self-directed change in their life.

Of course, clean language is not required or desirable in every clinical situation. For example, in an emergency the clinician must take charge, convey urgent need-to-know information, and provide needed opinion in response to direct questions or otherwise where required for the patient's welfare. Moreover, the language used in this situation is usually between healthcare professionals rather than with the patient. In contrast, clean language is particularly helpful when one needs to lead the patient to the solution. For example, in non-emergency settings, where it is desirable for a patient to take responsibility for lifestyle choices and where clear thinking on his or her part is required, consultations conducted in clean language may be more appropriate. Instead of statements and advice expressed in the doctor's words, clean language poses a series of questions using the patient's words to lead the patient to the understanding and solution. As the playwright Eugene Ionesco reputedly once said, and as many scientists will know, 'It is not the answer that enlightens, but the question.' As discussed in Chapter 7, humans try to make sense of their lives using metaphors, many of which are used subconsciously. Clean-language questions probe these metaphors as aids to understanding.[8]

No Claptrap

Low levels of health literacy are usually invoked when considering communication gaps between healthcare personnel and patients. Although awareness of health literacy can usefully direct attention toward the disadvantaged patient, loose use of the term often places the burden of responsibility on the patient rather than with the healthcare provider. The responsibility for ensuring that a patient understands the basic information needed to make appropriate health decisions lies with the carer. Consider the analogy with computer science, when it was commonplace to hear people refer to themselves as *computer-literate* or *computer-illiterate*. Had it remained that way, computer sales would never have skyrocketed. It quickly became apparent to the sellers of computers and software that the consumer will not buy or use their products if they can't use them. Today, all that is needed is the ability to plug in and switch on the computer. You don't even need to read the instruction manual. In some instances, everything can be done with touchscreen technology. Specialists can still deal in technical jargon, but the computer is useable by the everyman, and the term *computer-literacy* has become historic. Likewise, patients can't use health information in a sensible way if it is not made understandable.

After recovering from a serious illness, the poet Patrick Kavanagh was determined to record his gratitude 'without claptrap' ('for we must record love's mystery without claptrap'). By naming 'the common and banal' of the hospital ward, he was able to 'snatch out of time the passionate transitory'. Rows of cubicles, plain concrete, wash-basins, and even the fellow in the next bed, who snored, were included. The sonnet is testimony to the impact of simple language. There is no attempt to disguise or transform metaphorically the vernacular of the hospital paraphernalia. Direct, accessible language is used without sacrificing beauty, integrity or clarity. If this is possible in poetry, then the easier task of conveying ordinary healthcare messages without claptrap should be commonplace for experts.

How hard can it be? asks another poet, Elspeth Murray, in her plea for clarity of information to help patients trying to understand and make decisions regarding their illness. In a poem written for the launch of the cancer information reference group of SCAN, the South East Scotland Cancer Network (20 January 2006), she calls on the experts to 'speak like a human make it better not worse'. . . because illness is bad enough. The entire poem is reproduced here with the kind permission of Elspeth:

THIS IS BAD ENOUGH

This is bad enough
So please . . .
Don't give me
gobbledegook.

Don't give me
pages and dense pages
and
'this leaflet aims to explain . . . '

Don't give me
really dodgy photocopying
and
'DO NOT REMOVE
FOR REFERENCE ONLY.'

Don't give me
'*drafted in collaboration with
a multidisciplinary stakeholder
partnership consultation
short-life project working group.*'
I mean is this about
you guys
or me?

This is hard enough

So please:

Don't leave me
oddly none the wiser or
listening till my eyes are
glazing over.

Don't leave me
wondering what on earth that was about,
feeling like it's rude to ask
or consenting to goodness knows what.

Don't leave me
lost in another language
adrift in bad translation.

Don't leave me
chucking it in the bin
Don't leave me
leaving in the state I'm in.

Don't leave me
feeling even more clueless
than I did before any of this
happened.

This is tough enough
So please:

Make it relevant,
understandable –
or reasonably
readable
at least.

Why not put in
pictures
or sketches,
or something to
guide me through?

I mean how hard can it be
for the people
who are steeped in this stuff
to keep it up-to-date?

And you know what I'd appreciate?
A little time to take it in
a little time to show them at home
a little time to ask 'What's that?'
a little time to talk on the phone.

So give us
the clarity, right from the start
the contacts, there at the end.

Give us the info
you know we need to know.
Show us the facts,
some figures
And don't forget our feelings.

Because this is bad
and hard
and tough enough
so please speak
like a human
make it better
not worse.

—http://breastcancerconsortium.net/bad-enough-elspeth-
murray/

Social Media Medicine

When Jen Gunter needed information because her infant son had a
serious problem refluxing his feeds, she turned to the internet. Gunter
is a physician specialising in women's health, and knew how to access
authoritative medical websites. None of these sites met her needs,
however, in part because of the complexity of her son's heart and lung
problems, and in part because of her own emotional desperation. In the
end, she was drawn to websites where she 'felt understood' and which
used language that was 'intoxicating' in its 'confidence'. The problem with
those sites was that they were also selling products which were expensive
and useless. Fear sells. What she needed was 'sensible information from
a noted expert in a way that I could hear'. After more exploration, she
realised that her own patients were also encountering an internet of
misinformation and disinformation, and decided to write a textbook for
the public, with information that is clear and free of online distractions.

Tweets, hashtags, blogs, hangouts, podcasts and *wikis* may sound to an older generation like slang for bites and bed-bugs, but are in fact code for how a younger generation obtains health information. I don't counsel patients against using the internet or social media, but I do alert them to the lack of regulation in this area, and the difficulty of distinguishing truth from misinformation. Handled properly, social media can transform medical research, education and healthcare for the better. It is changing how patients interact with healthcare providers and the healthcare system. Social media may also be more democratic than traditional media, by delivering information to minority and lower socioeconomic groups with greater efficiency than traditional methods have done.

Access to information provides patients with a greater sense of control over their illness, but wisdom is still in short supply. In the words of Theodore Dalrymple, 'information without perspective is a higher form of ignorance'. For all their wonders, social technologies are not substitutes for human contact and the guiding help of doctors, nurses and other health professionals. Dissemination of misinformation, also a risk with traditional media, is accelerated on a vast scale by social media. 'A lie is halfway around the world before the truth has put its trousers on.' The spread of bad news and dangerous ideas on social media is like contagion. Ideas *go viral*, celebrities may become *super-spreaders*, and some social interactions favour the emergence of novel viruses with menacing names like *trojans, worms, ransomeware* and *malware*. Like infections, human behaviour makes false news spread more than truth online. This may be because humans have an overdramatic worldview, and are drawn to the fantastical more than to staid truths. As Gunter found, humans also tend to mistake repetition for accuracy – a problem amplified by retweets and reposts on social media.

6

⊰⊱⊰

No Words, Just Silent Signals

'like many another rare thing, the things that go unsaid are as valid
and meaningful as those that are said so beautifully.'
—Christy Brown[1]

*The Body Doesn't Lie – Small Behaviours – Looking the Part – Digital
Doc and the Third Presence – The Most Under-rated Clinical Discipline
– The Importance of Silences – Doctoring as a Performance Art – Style –
Touching – Presence – An Important Resource*

Patients and carers use more than words to interact. Effective
communicators don't have to say much – sometimes nothing at
all. When I was in my internship, the first year after graduating from
medical school, I worked under the supervision of an experienced
clinician who was notorious for his silences. The team learned to stay
quiet in his presence. We would conduct ward-rounds that were serene,
sailing silently in and out of the hospital wards. His routine was to sit
at the bedside of each patient under his care. His salutation was a nod
or a smile. While sitting, he would hold the patient's wrist, feeling the
pulse, even though we could all see the telemetry tracings of the vital
signs over the patient's head. That wasn't the point. He was making
contact with the patient without words. He would listen to the progress
report while observing the patient, grunt or grimace a little, and then
nod reassuringly again to the patient, as if to say: 'Yes, all is in order
here.' Then, we would sail on in silence. Afterwards, I would relay to
the nurses that the boss wanted them to do this-this-this-and-that,
to which they would often respond with a puzzled look: 'You mean
you actually heard him say all of that?' After he retired, one of his
colleagues remarked that he never used one word when none would do.

The subtlety of silent signalling was beautifully recounted by Dr
Kimberly Manning, a black hospital-based clinician in Atlanta, who
described in the *Journal of the American Medical Association* something

remarkable from an otherwise ordinary ward-round that she had conducted. The parade led by Dr Manning along the hospital corridors, in and out of different wards, with a posse of culturally and ethnically diverse students, would not have appeared unusual. She did this every day. Then, one of the students, who seemed to scrutinise her every move, was curious as to how Dr Manning seemed to know so many of the people that they had passed on the ward-round. The keen young student had noticed a series of almost imperceptible salutations, gestures or acknowledgements exchanged between Dr Manning and a miscellany of strangers, nurses, porters, patients and visitors, none of whom were participants in the ward-round. The student had sensed 'one of the most universal yet untaught gestures of black American culture: "the nod",' a tiny dip of the head whereby two members of a minority acknowledge each other. The author Anatole Broyard also noted beauty in the unspoken 'signing' exchanged between two strangers of similar ethnicity when passing in the street.

I had witnessed something similar during my fellowship in gastroenterology at the University of California, Los Angeles. There was a remarkable man who ran the endoscopy unit at the Wadsworth Veterans Administration hospital at the time, Mr D. He was patient with the trainees and rarely said no. He was hard working, kind, and a dedicated servant to the patients. He stood tall and dignified at all times, and he was black. The fellows were from all over the world, and all were white Caucasian, as were almost all of the attending physicians. One of the visiting gastroenterologists, who came about once a month to conduct a teaching session with us, was black. Although Mr D treated everyone the same way, there was something ever-so-slightly special about his greeting with that visiting endoscopist.

The subtle signal of acknowledgement is not unique to black American culture. It's how we send the message: 'I see you.' There is something quite beautiful about this, an instinctive nod, the unconscious gesture, which Dr Manning rightly feels is more likely to unify than polarise, grants access to what she describes as 'our cultural mysteries', and ultimately improves communication between doctors and patients, and with each other.

THE BODY DOESN'T LIE

Humans use language skills for communicating ideas of subtlety or complexity, for communicating at distance and, sadly, for manipulation of the truth. Animals can communicate and cooperate with one another without language, but so also do humans. Indeed, most human-to-human signals are non-verbal. Non-verbal communication may be speech-related (tone of voice, speaking time, interruptions) or speech-unrelated through body language (facial expression, stance, gazing, nodding, eye-contact, posture, gestures, interpersonal distance, dress, positional orientation relative to patient).

Non-verbal communication is a means of signalling rejection or sexual attraction. Mae West, the controversial sex-symbol of the American Depression era, and famous for her double entrendres, once said: 'I speak two languages, Body and English.' Not surprisingly, most of the great writers and thinkers were alert to the power of non-verbal cues.

> Fie, fie upon her!
> There's language in her eye, her cheek, her lip,
> Nay, her foot speaks; her wanton spirits look out
> At every joint and motive of her body
> —William Shakespeare, *Troilus and Cressida,* Act IV, Scene V

However, most non-verbal communication operates at a sub-conscious level. In contrast to verbal language and word-choice, humans have less control over non-verbal signals. The American dance choreographer Martha Graham believed that the body never lies: 'To me, the body says what words cannot . . . . That doesn't mean that it's telling a story, but it means it's communicating a feeling, a sensation to people.'

We can speak with flattery or forked tongue, but find it more difficult to conceal the truth with non-verbal communication. Once again, Shakespeare had something to say about this. In *Macbeth* (I, 4, 13-14), the king naively thinks: 'There's no art/ To find the mind's construction in the face' but Macbeth later acknowledges that 'False face must hide what the false heart doth know' when goaded by Lady Macbeth: 'Your face, my thane, is a book where men/ May read strange matters . . . look like the innocent flower.'

Doctors have always been aware of non-verbal cues from their patients, and continually assess sickness-behaviour. Experienced clinicians know the 'sick look', and are continually vigilant for it. Observing patients while they wait, or as they walk from the waiting area to the interview room, will frequently alert the astute clinician that something is amiss, regardless of what the patient says. Hesitancy in responding to certain questions, a glance away, a tear, a change in facial expression, or a simple gesture may be more revealing than the verbal responses in the medical interview. This form of communication is two-directional, and it is self-evident that conscientious clinicians should consider how their own non-verbal signals are interpreted by the patient. In particular, when non-verbal cues from a doctor conflict with the verbal, the former will usually override the latter, and lead to doubt or distrust of what the doctor is telling the patient. The consequences include dissatisfaction with the medical interview, loss of confidence, and poor adherence by the patient to medical advice.

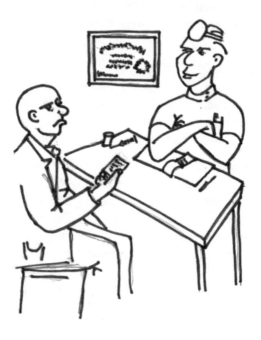

Look at the image above. The body language of doctor and patient are strikingly different. This is clearly an asymmetric relationship. No one would have difficulty identifying which one is in crisis, and for which one the encounter is routine.

SMALL BEHAVIOURS

In studying face-to-face interactions, the legendary sociologist Erving Goffman referred to the small behaviours which are continuously active, and which shape the outcome of the medical encounter – whether intended or not. Tiny details of the physician's behaviour are detected by a patient. Small gestures, glances and positioning assume enhanced significance for a patient in crisis. Confident people use more space than non-confident people. This allows doctors to project an air of confidence and reassurance by body-language alone.

'What casual gestures these doctors are permitted!' a mother thinks to herself as the oncologist hurriedly presents treatment options with a casual shrug In Lorrie Moore's story of childhood cancer. Acutely sensitised, the mother notices minute details and thinks to herself: 'He is a skilled manual labourer. The tricky emotional stuff is not to his liking.'

Experienced clinicians are self-aware and conscious not to display the casualness of the routine. Dr Roger Kneebone has actually likened the skilled clinician to a magician in close-up live performance, who is continually and consciously managing subtle signals and responses to and from the audience. First impressions for the patient happen within seconds. In an article entitled 'The Three-second Consultation', Dr John Launer described his study of video recordings of doctor-patient consultations, during which he was drawn to tiny details of the doctors' behaviour within the first three seconds of the patient entering the interview room. Before the first question, the movement, gestures and facial expression of the doctor created a welcoming feeling, and a momentary pause enabled the patient to compose him- or herself. Likewise, from the physician's perspective, I believe it is a lost opportunity not to observe the patient before the consultation begins. By greeting the patient in the waiting area, there is valuable non-verbal information to be sensed from the patient's mood, demeanour and movement in walking from the waiting room to the interview room.

Common errors of non-verbal communication can be avoided or minimised by simple good manners and kindness. A yawn is inexcusable. Anything other than close listening is unacceptable. Indeed, much of what passes for a doctor's communication skills is within the realm of common sense and politeness. The small behaviours of eye-contact, facial expression, posture, positioning and proximity are particularly important when dealing with the elderly, the deaf, and depressed and anxious patients, but they are paramount when giving bad news.

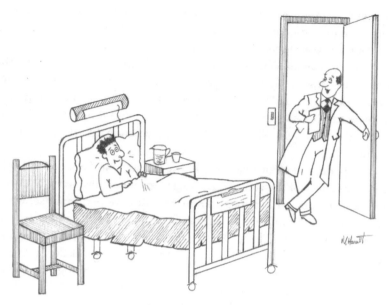

'How are we today? I'll have someone pop by when the test results are back,
and I'll see you as an outpatient in six weeks.'
The body-language and words of a man wishing to be elsewhere.

LOOKING THE PART

It is not difficult to find popular books and magazine articles that tell us
that our clothes influence how we think, and that what we wear is a form
of non-verbal communication. Doctors and patients dress differently.
This at once reflects the asymmetric nature of their relationship, and
conforms to the different roles they play in the illness drama, but it may
also be a means by which they judge each other. *Thin-slicing*, a term
used in popular psychology books, refers to judgements made on the
basis of momentary glimpses (thin slices) of information. The concept
was popularised by Malcolm Gladwell in his book *Blink*. These narrow
slices of information embody first impressions and are prone to error,
but doctors and patients unconsciously and continually thin-slice each
other.

Doctors are trained to use all of their senses when assessing
patients. It begins with inspection and attention to detail, including
inspection of the patient's surroundings at the bedside. But details
are only informative when considered in context and measured, not
overstated. An ashtray in the wrong place or a bag full of medications at

the bedside may or may not be informative, and the presence of tattoos or nail-varnish on the toenails does not necessarily imply anything risqué about the patient's lifestyle. One of the elderly clinicians who taught me while I was training used to say that women who were jaundiced tended to wear pastel shades of yellow, and those who had respiratory disease tended to wear shades of blue, to camouflage their cyanotic discolouration. I doubt this was based on evidential fact, and never found it helpful, but patients do send non-verbal signals to their doctor in other ways. For example, outpatients may display car keys or a parking ticket in hand, representing impatience, pressure of time or, more usually, the importance of their lives outside the context of the doctor-patient interaction. In hospital, patients may unwittingly resist playing the sick role by sitting beside – not *in* – their bed during daytime, and by wearing their work clothes rather than pyjamas. For me, this is seldom evidence of absent illness, but rather it enhances the urgency of restoring the patient to health, and back to their real-world life outside the hospital. These subtle signals offset the dominance of the caregiver, and restore the centrality of the patient.

If clothing is a form of non-verbal signalling, it is two-directional. Time slows down when people are sick, and they note the finest of details worn by their doctors. A dramatic example of this occurs in the first episode of the popular TV series *Breaking Bad* (2008-13), in which the protagonist Walter White is told he has end-stage lung cancer. 'Do you understand what I've just told you?' asks his doctor, to whom Walter responds: 'Yes. Lung cancer. Inoperable. It's just you've got this mustard stain on your shirt.' Stunned and stressed, he understands, but his focus on the sloppiness of the doctor's clothing signals a momentary doctor-patient disconnect.

People seldom admit that they draw inferences or judge doctors based on their clothing. When patients are surveyed, they seldom concede that they have an opinion on appropriate or desirable clothing for their doctor, and usually declare this to be unimportant, or at least rank it well below other factors, such as kindness, competence and attitude. For Nassim Nicholas Taleb, who has written extensively on life's uncertainties, surgeons should not look like surgeons. Faced with a choice of two surgeons of equal rank, one who looks the part and could play the part in a movie, the other looking more like an overweight and unkempt butcher, he would choose the latter. His reason? In achieving some measure of success, those who don't look the part are likely to have overcome more, and overcoming perception is likely to have filtered out incompetence. Taleb is correct that true expertise is blind to appearances, but many will find his case for selecting a surgeon based on this concept alone, unconvincing. A contrarian view was taken by Dr David Mendel in *Proper Doctoring,* a book for patients and their doctors. 'The patient's point of view must prevail,' argued Mendel. Moreover, it is the point of view of the most conventionally minded patient who must determine the way a doctor should look. Regardless of how brilliant a doctor may be, eccentric clothes and hairdos should be avoided; nasal studs and loud Hawaiian shirts are unlikely to inspire confidence in elderly, frightened patients. After general appearances, patients usually observe the hands of a doctor touching them – with the reasonable expectation of cleanliness.

DIGITAL DOC AND THE THIRD PRESENCE

A few years ago, a large colour image was published in the *Journal of the American Medical Association,* which showed a doctor-patient interaction in a consulting room through the eyes of a seven-year-old girl.[2] The doctor, referred to by one of his colleagues as someone who 'delivers humanity with competence', was probably in regular receipt of colourful drawings from his young patients. But this one was different, and disturbing. The artist was the seven-year-old patient sitting smiling on the exam table, with her mother holding her baby sister and an older sister nearby. A smiling, happy scene, but with one big problem: the doctor had his back to the patient and her family, and was focused attentively on his computer-screen. The associated commentary addressed the distancing or dehumanising effect of technology, and the new reality of the computer as a 'third player' in the patient-doctor relationship.

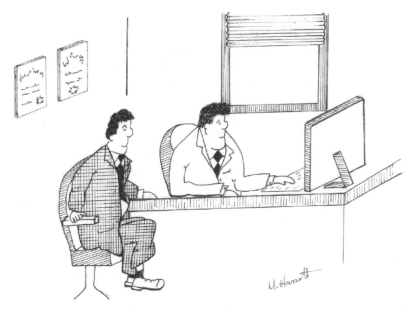

The third presence

There are ways to reduce the distracting influence of the digital third presence which help rehumanise the consultation. Firstly, the screen should be shared with the patient. Alternatively, voice-recognition devices can free the doctor from having to spend time typing onto the electronic health-record. Better again would be the employment of a human scribes to record the essentials while the clinician focuses on the patient. Unless some action is taken, *digital doctors* offer little more than can be achieved with a touchscreen and may, in effect, be typing themselves out of a job.

THE MOST UNDERRATED CLINICAL DISCIPLINE

Listening. To develop an ear for the difference between what people feel and what they say, one must listen. When you're talking, you're not listening. In every story, that which is left unsaid is sometimes more important than what has been made explicit. Consider the lean prose of James Joyce and the effect created by a series of unfinished sentences in the short story 'The Sisters' from the *Dubliners* collection. The story is narrated by a young boy who is trying to make sense of the death of a defrocked priest, his friend and mentor. Fragments of dialogue overheard by the boy suggest that the boy-priest relationship may have been something less than wholesome: 'No, I wouldn't say he was exactly . . . but there was something queer . . . there was something uncanny about him . . . ', 'I think it was one of those . . . peculiar cases . . . But it's hard to say . . . ' and 'I wouldn't like children of mine . . . to have much to say to a man like that.'

Like Joyce, Arthur Conan Doyle had received medical training, and understood the importance of the negative observation. Something which is neither seen nor heard is the key to his story of Sherlock Holmes and Silver Blaze. When Holmes is asked by the local police if there was any point to which he wished to draw their attention, Holmes responded: 'To the curious incident of the dog in the night-time.' 'The dog did nothing in the night-time', said Inspector Gregory. 'That,' said Holmes, 'was the curious incident.'

Listening is an essential skill for success in all forms of human interaction. 'The most important thing in communication is hearing what isn't said,' according to Peter Drucker, the much-quoted leadership and management guru. Entrepreneur Bill Liao identifies different kinds of listening. First, there are those who wait to speak: they wait for the gap in conversation to make their point, without actually responding to what has already been said. Second, are those who listen to judge: they are forming a judgement as one speaks, without waiting to hear the full dialogue. Third, are the sympathy listeners. These people give the appearance of listening: they maintain eye-contact, but are not attentively listening. Finally, there is listening to re-create. These people listen with ears and eyes to develop understanding or empathy with what the speaker is saying, and suspend judgement until they have heard the speaker in full. As in business, a successful doctor-patient consultation needs the latter form of listening from both participants.

The Importance of Silences

Silence is a valuable device in interviews. People feel a need to fill silences, but it should be the interviewee, rather than the interviewer, who fills the silence. Inexperienced interviewers cannot resist the urge to bridge a silence by asking a question. Strategic silence was one of the tricks of the trade for Robert Caro, a multiple-award-winning investigative journalist, famous for his meticulous biography of US president Lyndon B. Johnson. When he sensed that an interviewee might divulge a sensitive piece of information unasked for, he would jot down a note to himself: 'SU' (for Shut Up!). Caro acclaims two of the greatest fictional detectives, Georges Simenon's Inspector Maigret and John le Carré's George Smiley, for their deliberate use of silence in interviews. Tension mounted when Maigret paused to clean his pipe, provoking the witness to nervously blurt out more information, whereas Smiley would remove his spectacles to polish them with the end of his necktie, waiting for the witness to break down.

Silence is, of itself, part of effective doctor-patient communication. As discussed above, effective listening requires discipline; it is an active not a passive process, distinct from waiting to speak. This distinction has been lost on many of the politicians and other talking-heads on television and radio, whose only pause is to ready themselves to speak again, rather than actively listen.

An old aphorism goes as follows: 'Sometimes it is better to look foolish and say nothing than to open your mouth and remove all doubt.' This may be sound advice for students and trainees, and occasional politicians, who have no sensible answer or explanation to give. But effective doctors have also learnt from experience how to sense when they should say nothing. Patients do not always seek tests, drugs or easy solutions. Some just need to tell their story and be listened to. A satisfactory consultation can often be achieved by simply granting the patient the courtesy of an attentive hearing.

There is nothing new here; listening to the patient's story is the essence of narrative medicine as championed by Rita Charon and others. An illness-story told in a patient's own words does not consume an inordinate amount of time. In fact, most studies have found that giving the patient time to speak consumes far less time than many clinicians estimate.

On numerous occasions, I have been referred patients who have already exhausted all other medical opinions, had all the usual tests and been prescribed countless, ineffective remedies. The consultation often begins with the patient saying: 'Doctor, you're my last hope.' Most experienced clinicians will recognise the familiar scenario. This is what some have described as a 'heart-sink' patient: the kind who seems unhappy, is likely to take up a lot of time, and is unlikely to be satisfied with the consultation. Time invested during the initial consultation with this patient is cost-effective. It is what Margaret McCartney, in her book *The Patient Paradox,* has termed the 'small significances' and the 'quiet side of medicine'. In fact, this is the kind of patient most likely to benefit from a respectful hearing and heartfelt gestures of compassion. I like to think of it as prescribing time in divided doses. The initial dose may seem to be large, but it will make subsequent exchanges with the patient more efficient, and will transform what might have seemed to be a tedious encounter into an effective and gratifying one.

When doctors recount patients' stories of elusive diagnoses, there is invariably one case where the diagnosis is arrived at because the doctor remains silent. A favourite is that described by Dr David Watts, an American gastroenterologist and frequent contributor to literature on medical humanities. He acknowledges that the traditional diagnostician is portrayed like a latter-day Sherlock Holmes, who assembles the key facts extracted from the patient under direct questioning, and proceeds with linear multi-step logic to a conclusive solution. However, illness is not like a detective drama. It is more akin to theatre of the absurd. It is abstract and sometimes irrational. The story Watts tells is one in which, by his silence, he encouraged his patient to speak and arrive at a conclusion as to what was really bothering her. 'I think you needed a place where it was possible to hear yourself talk. When it was quiet enough . . . you heard the answer.' Her chronic symptoms did not need drugs; the solution was evident once a domestic problem had been acknowledged.

Doctoring as a Performance Art

Dr Michael O'Donnell, the popular broadcaster, editor of the journal *World Medicine* and author of numerous books on doctoring, observed that his father, a family practitioner in England, changed his behaviour and became a performer in the presence of patients. The young O'Donnell noticed, when accompanying his father on house-calls, that the older doctor would modify his act according to the nature of the patient's clinical problem. In the same way that a performing artist senses the mood of the audience, good doctors acquire an ability to see things as they appear to the eyes of their patient. This, concluded O'Donnell, is where empathy begins.

To be convincing, not phoney, the doctor's performance, like that of an actor, must embody integrity and be truthful to his or her own self. For O'Donnell, the doctor's performance is creative; in that respect it differs from role-playing and bedside manner. He has criticised the time spent on teaching self-evident truths and much of what passes for training in medical communication skills, which he and others have found to be banal. John Skelton, a professor of clinical communication in the UK, has warned that more attention needs to be given to the attitude of doctors to their different roles, rather than reducing communication to the mechanics of role-playing and the use of stock phrases or formulaic techniques. As with drama students, it may be more fruitful if doctors were encouraged to learn more about themselves and their attitude to patients and to professional life, rather than concentrating exclusively on the techniques of communication.

Doctors dislike the word 'acting' as a descriptor for their interaction with patients, but have no difficulty casting patients in a sick role. Doctors tend to prefer words like 'professionalism', for fear that the A-word implies some form of cynicism or callousness. Others have argued that patients are particularly concerned with a doctor's attitude, which is conveyed in both verbal and non-verbal messages. The influential sociologist Erving Goffman acknowledged with a nod toward Shakespeare that 'All the world is not, of course, a stage, but the crucial ways in which it isn't are not easy to specify'. Doctors need to be able to act as if they care, even when harbouring a dislike for a patient – which they must know how to mask. An ability to show concern for a patient's distress requires non-verbal as well as verbal self-awareness. Even when harried and tired at the end of a busy day, and regardless of their mood, gifted doctors can adapt their behaviour to respond to a patient's concerns. In this context, acting is not a deception; it is a willingness to act out one's personality.[3] This requires practice, coaching and self-reflection. While primarily intended for the patients welfare, the doctor can also benefit from this form of acting because it turns the ordinary into the extraordinary, and renders enjoyable what might otherwise be jaded or routine. In so doing, it makes the doctor less vulnerable to the modern pandemic of 'burnout'.

STYLE

'My urologist is a very handsome man . . . he comes into the room like a bullfighter. He has style. He has magic and is extremely competent. He doesn't talk. He's too much of a star, but he has an oncologist who talks for him.' This description is from Anatole Broyard's quirky memoir.

Style, according to psychologists, is about how one engages with and presents oneself to the world. It reflects self-confidence and attitude. It is individual. A doctor's style was more influential in the past, when the scientific basis of medicine was weak, and doctors had limited capacity to cure their patients. The description by Marcel Proust of the non-fictional Dr Georges Dieulafoy, who had been sent for, not to cure but to certify the gravity of his grandmother's illness, is illustrative. 'To the dignity of his bearing was added, without being conspicuous, the litheness of a perfect figure . . . decorum suited to distressing circumstances . . . . In the sable majesty of his frock-coat, the Professor would enter the room, melancholy without affectation, uttering not one word of condolence that could have been construed as insincere, not being guilty of the slightest infringement of the rules of tact.' After skilfully examining the patient, the eminent doctor, who was 'the embodiment of tact, intelligence and kindness', made a perfect exit – but not before accepting his fee in the sealed envelope that was slipped into his hand, which he made vanish with a 'conjuror's dexterity . . . without sacrificing one iota of gravity'.

Attitude is the element of style that modern patients care most about in their doctor. Other things are, of course, important, but none more so than attitude. Dr Bernard Lown, renowned cardiologist and Nobel Peace Prize winner, noticed that as he got older, patients continued to cling to him, even though his technical expertise had declined. He concluded that what patients wanted was a doctor who understood and was interested in them. Likewise for Anatole Broyard, it was important that the doctor know that he was more than his illness: 'I wouldn't demand a lot of my doctor's time: I just wish he would . . . give me his whole mind just once.' Broyard wanted his doctor to be interested in him, and for him to be interested in the doctor. While the doctor 'inevitably feels superior to me,' he wrote, 'I'd like him to know that I feel superior to him', and wished that there could be a place where their respective superiorities could 'meet and frolic together'.

TOUCHING

Imagine what it might be like to never touch or be touched, skin on skin. Infants need handling to thrive, the grief-stricken need a hug, and the sick heal under the influence of a caregiver's hand. The importance of contact by touching is reflected in the language we use: we are 'touched' by deep emotions, sense the tension as 'palpable', dislike being 'rubbed up the wrong way' and need to stay 'in touch' with our doctors. Will this be fundamentally altered post-Covid? Loss of direct human contact adds to the suffering during an outbreak of infection. However, even during the Covid-19 pandemic, the human impulse to touch was retained, with hands placed on either side of glass barriers separating visitors from cocooned loved ones.

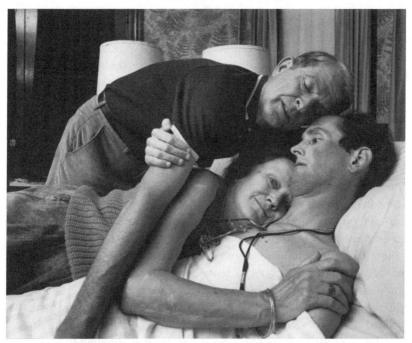

Robert Sappenfield and His Parents, Dorchester, Massachusetts, 1988
© Nicholas Nixon, courtesy Fraenkel Gallery, San Francisco

Helen Keller, who was blind and deaf from an early age, wrote a stirring testimony for the power of human touch: how much it could tell her about the world around her and of 'the warmth and protectiveness of the hand'. Although the senses assist and reinforce one another, 'touch is a great deal the eye's superior', she wrote, and 'I would not part with the warm, endearing contact of human hands or the wealth of form, the mobility and fullness that press into my palms'.

The laying-on of hands is the oldest skill in doctoring. Once, it conferred a magic-like quality on doctors when they had little else to offer patients. Later, palpation and percussion became core diagnostic skills, whereas today touching has a different value. As a diagnostic instrument, the physical examination is subordinate to the patient's story, and while the changing role of the physical examination is conceded, its value is consistently upheld in commentaries on doctoring by experts such as Lewis Thomas, Bernard Lown, Roger Kneebone, Richard. B. Weinberg and Danielle Ofri. The physical examination does more than gather tactile information; it is a moment of silence. Often, it is the period when patients relax and reveal what is bothering them most.

Doctors through the ages have used the physical examination as a moment to probe non-medical as well as medical issues which may be bothering their patients. Although doctors were seldom portrayed favourably in Victorian novels, an exception was the hero in Trollope's *Dr Thorne*, whose skill was to draw on all of his senses in making an astute and holistic assessment of his patients. When dealing with a privileged but difficult patient, 'The doctor, in the meantime, had taken Sir Roger's hand on the pretext of feeling his pulse, but drawing quite as much information from the touch of the sick man's skin, and the look of the sick man's eye.'

For many patients, a physical examination is an expected part of the consultation, and they may feel that their symptoms are not taken seriously if it is not part of the consultation. ('He didn't even bother to examine me.') For others, disrobing and submitting the semi-naked body to examination by a stranger may be traumatic, even humiliating, particularly for younger patients. Lucy Grealy described feeling 'humiliated and exposed' when asked to strip down while the doctor talked to the nurse, her mother and someone on the phone which was tucked beneath his chin. The 'gruff' doctor, she recalls, 'spoke far too loudly', 'prodded' her with his hands, 'hit me just slightly too hard' with his reflex-hammer, drew blood from a vein after tying the tourniquet too tightly.

Humans, like other animals, subconsciously protect their personal space and feel vulnerable, uncomfortable or threatened if this peri-personal space is encroached. In his 2018 book *The Spaces Between Us*, neuroscientist Michael Graziano describes the medical and social implications of personal space and how it is monitored in the brain. Skilful clinicians respect a patient's personal space. They know when and when not to navigate that space. They invest time and care with no little skill to ensure that the physical examination is unfussy, gentle and without discomfort.

The experienced clinician also knows that the laying-on of hands is an opportunity to realise the value of touch. Touch as a nonverbal form of expression is underestimated by many, and seldom taught. Touch can convey confidence, authority, reassurance and competency, or, if it is tentative and awkward, it can foster doubt. No fumbling, or the effect is lost. It begins with the handshake, the quality of which assumes particular importance when the distancing effect of ritual handwashing, gloves and gown-ups are required. Danielle Ofri occasionally resorts to the clinical examination if she feels that the interview with a patient is at an impasse or has reached an awkward stage. In other words, non-verbal communication by touching can compensate or make up for the challenges that may arise in a patient-doctor interaction.

Dr Richard Horton, editor of the medical journal the *Lancet,* was a medical student in the 1980s but was surprised to find in contemporary clinical practice that the physical examination has become an anachronism, largely replaced by high-tech investigations. 'Who needs doctors?' he asks, and comments that their role has become 'ambiguous'. 'The avoidance of touch is bad medicine', claims Horton, and quotes the popular author Margaret Atwood, who wrote in *The Blind Assassin* (2000): 'Touch comes before sight, before speech, it is the first language and the last, and it always tells the truth.' Touch fosters a sense of connection between doctor and patient, and builds trust and reassurance.

Presence

Presence is the soul of caring. Presence, as defined by Dr Arthur Kleinman, is the 'intensity of interacting with another human being that animates being there for, and with, that person.' Presence is an active rather than passive demonstration that one's humanity matters to another.

There is a story from World War I, in which a soldier found himself dazed in a shelled-out crater on the battlefield. When the dust settled and the smoke receded, he realised he was not alone. An enemy soldier lay opposite him. Immediately, they squared up with rifle and bayonet, but then, something extraordinary happened. Their eyes met. They paused, a moment passed, and they quietly left the crater in opposite directions. That was presence.

In another story, the playwright Alan Bennett recalled being in agony with unrelieved pain in hospital, while the medics were preoccupied with inserting a tube into his abdomen to drain an abscess. A passer-by in the corridor paused and squeezed Bennett's hand until relief arrived, and the abscess was located and drained. Then, the stranger patted the hand and continued away. 'This uncalled-for gesture was perhaps the kindest thing anyone had ever done for me.' This kindness was a moment of presence.

Presence doesn't depend on words, just authentic engagement, feeling and listening. For Kleinman, the most memorable aspects of his fifty-year-long career have been occasions of presence which have sustained him and helped prevent burnout: being a clinician 'liberated me from inveterate personality faults. It taught me a great lesson in humanity. It has enriched and deepened my life experience. Not least it made me more present to others and to myself.'

AN IMPORTANT RESOURCE

Many doctors will avoid contact when it appears that there is little more that they can offer their patient. Testimony from patients reveals that this is when the doctor is most needed. I recall the wisdom of an old clinician telling me of an older clinician who used to ask the young doctors: 'What is the most important resource in the hospital available to you when you have a patient for whom there are no treatment options left?' Usual responses include mute, blank stares or vague suggestions about consultations with palliative medicine or the chaplain. Correct answer: the bedside chair.

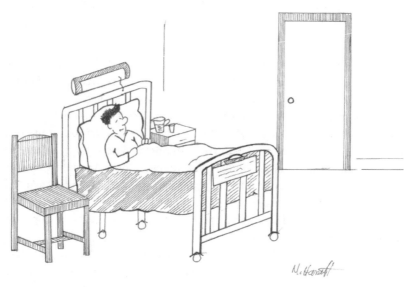

The bedside chair: an important therapeutic resource

7

Healing Words, Hurting Words

'Words! Mere words! How terrible they were! How clear, and vivid, and cruel! One could not escape from them. And yet what a subtle magic there was in them!

—Oscar Wilde, *The Picture of Dorian Gray*

The Barracuda at the Front Office – Dr Nocebo and Dr Placebo – Metaphoric Medic – Who's Afraid of Susan Sontag? – The Personal Metaphor – Dappled Things – Sticks and Stones . . . and Stigma – Stigma Stories from Sick Doctors – Science and Stigma – Tell It Slant

If doctors can help just by listening, and if they can soothe with kind words, they can also hurt and harm with poorly chosen words. In 1934, the renowned medical scientist Dr Lawrence J. Henderson warned young doctors at the Harvard Medical School Colloquium as follows: 'In your relations with your patients you will inevitably do much harm, and this will be by no means confined to your strictly medical blunders. It will arise also from what you say and what you fail to say.' Sixty years later, cardiologist and winner of the Nobel Prize for Peace Dr Bernard Lown was writing: 'Words are the most powerful tool a doctor possesses, but words, like a two-edged sword, can maim as well as heal.' This captures the concept of the doctor-as-drug: usually beneficial, occasionally with adverse effects.

Regardless of how well a doctor may be coached in communication skills, the patient's experience is the measure of outcome. A good patient-doctor consultation differs from a bad one in how it makes the patient feel. As outlined in the introductory chapter 'When Crisis Meets Routine', the patient-doctor relationship is at first uneven, beset with multiple asymmetries. Over time, the physician's ability to foster confidence and trust by redressing such imbalances determines the outcome for the patient.

The medical consultation begins, like other human encounters, with first impressions. Doctors are trained to be aware of the powerful impact of first impressions on human judgement and on subsequent decision-making, referred to as *anchoring bias*. The anchoring effect was defined by the studies of the late Amos Tversky and Nobel laureate Daniel Kahnemann. Anchoring effects occur subconsciously, are difficult to avoid, but are important to be wary of, because a doctor's first impressions of a patient's symptoms may impact on his or her ability to make an accurate diagnosis or to decide on a course of treatment suited to the patient. Anchoring works both ways; patients are like all humans: hard-wired to make quick judgements of people – including their doctors and other healthcare professionals.

First Impressions: The Barracuda at the Front Office

Doctors only get one chance to make a good first impression when consulted by a patient. First impressions are made up of small things. Small things count. The following vignette is a true account that I jotted down after I accompanied my son for a consultation with a world-leading expert. Joe, my son, the patient, had a serious illness. I was his support, and I was the one who was terrified. Joe didn't say much, but this is what I thought about the consultation[1]:

> Eyes smiling, face beaming, the porter rose from his stool to greet arrivals at the cancer centre, each nervously hesitant, staying close to a supporting loved one. With the confidence of a man who enjoyed being good at his job, he paused for those needing directions, reassured us that we were in the right place for our appointment, and then boomed: 'Welcome everyone, and good luck to you all today.'
>
> Good start. After that, we didn't mind inconveniences like waiting for the single working elevator, and felt better about whatever unknowns were ahead. The moment was still fresh when we got to the sixth floor. There, we faced a receptionist unable to switch her gaze from a computer to address us. Detached, with jaded eyes fixed elsewhere, her outstretched arm dispatched us to an adjacent touchscreen to register. We obeyed but the system insisted on a five-digit address code. Bad enough to be labelled 'international' as code for not having acceptable insurance, but not having a zip-code was a new stigma. Before we could explain, Miss No-Eye-Contact was on

the phone staring at some distant point behind us, then back to her screen with a facial expression that said: 'Can't you see! I'm busy.' Bristling a little, I blurted out my son's details to demand attention. Without the slightest shift in posture, she confirmed our existence in the system with a few flicks of her keyboard. Progress. Then she left us with the unsettling comment: 'Hmm, that's interesting . . . take a seat and wait while I check with Accounts.' This is not what patients want to hear as they contemplate the prospect of major surgery. No one wants to be that kind of interesting.

Joe shot a warning glance at me. 'Dad . . . don't be rude with this lady. Don't lose it!'

Lose it! After eight months of continual worry and stress trying to steer my son through the complexities and decision-making of a young man's cancer treatment, I was determined not to 'lose it'. We were overseas in a different healthcare system for a high-stakes operation. They were now in charge, and I would just have to play it their way. After all, I wasn't the patient. I was supposed to be the support. So I stayed quiet. Then, the silence was broken, delightfully so, it seemed to me, when an old woman behind us flatly refused to have anything to do with self-registration. Dismissing the technology with an impatient wave of her hand, she snapped at no one in particular in a brash accent: 'I'm not gonna do it, I can't be bothered with that.'

Miss No-Eye-Contact receptionist had met her match.

While waiting, I imagined myself telling anyone seeking my opinion that professional staff within medical offices and hospitals should heed the little things that comfort patients. I would tell them that little things are important. Staff should know that routine for them is crisis for the patient. I would remind them that there is only one opportunity to make a first impression. First impressions are made up of little things. Little things can make a big impression. If the front-office experience is poor, anxiety increases, and confidence in the rest of the enterprise becomes more doubtful. In other words, if the dentist's receptionist is a barracuda, don't expect much pain relief when you get to the back-office.

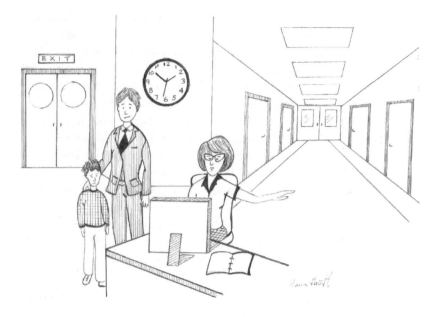

Then, we heard our name called out and we were on our way into the back office.

The interview with the surgeon was probably over within minutes but it seemed much longer. He began with a firm handshake. Then, sitting beside us, not across a table, he spoke confidently in clear, crisp, explanatory sentences. These, he must have repeated on hundreds of previous occasions, but it didn't seem that way. He anticipated our questions and acknowledged our sense of urgency.

In the end, the professionalism of the porter that morning, and his memorable welcome, was the bellwether for what followed. The surgeon's skill and experienced team determined what was to be a favourable outcome. But something else made a difference, and a lasting impression. To borrow from the poet Maya Angelou: 'people will forget what you said, people will forget what you did, but people will never forget how you made them feel'.

Dr Nocebo and Dr Placebo

Every treatment is modified either positively (placebo effect) or negatively (nocebo) by the quality of doctor-patient communication. Writing in the *Lancet* medical journal more than thirty years ago, the neurologist Dr

J N Blau advised that 'the doctor who fails to have a placebo effect on his patients should become a pathologist or an anaesthetist . . . If the patient does not feel better for your consultation you are in the wrong game.' The same career guidance applies to doctors who unwittingly convey nocebo effects to their patients.

While the placebo effect is a continual source of fascination for clinicians and scientists, the nocebo effect has received much less attention. As originally used, the term 'nocebo' refers to the undesirable effects of inert or sham medications: the negative equivalent, or opposite, of placebo effects. Nocebo is now used in a wider context to encompass unwanted new or worsening symptoms due to negative expectations or unintended negative cues from the doctor or nurse. The implication of placebo and nocebo phenomena for routine daily clinical practice relates to a doctor's skill in using words and non-verbal cues which, as alluded to earlier, enhance rather than diminish the intended effects of prescribed treatments.

Routine communication skills are uncomplicated and generally fall within the realm of common sense. Most doctors have common sense but don't always apply it. Self-awareness, curiosity and continual self-questioning can sensitise doctors and nurses to the nocebo and placebo impact of their words. Likewise, patients in crisis are hypersensitive, anxious, and susceptible to positive and negative suggestion, and at risk of becoming hazard-fixated. The doctor's choice of words may offset or escalate these problems. Use of positive words and healing imagery is preferable to negative and painful imagery. For example, it is clearly preferable to tell a patient that local anaesthetic will *numb* the area rather than saying 'This will *sting* a bit but will reduce the *pain*.' In addition, when prescription of a drug or new treatment is accompanied by a confident positive recommendation, the outcome is likely to be more satisfactory than if the recommendation is ambiguous and vague. No marks for guessing whether the following prescriptions are from Dr Placebo or Dr Nocebo: 'I dunno if these pills are any good, but I know a guy who says they might be' and 'This is gonna hurt like hell, so go ahead and have a good scream now and get it over with!'

METAPHORIC MEDIC

Everyone is familiar with the use of metaphors to enliven and provide colour in literary works. 'History is a nightmare from which I'm trying to awake' James Joyce famously wrote in *A Portrait of the Artist as a Young Man*, whereas 'an aged man is but a paltry thing, a tattered coat upon a stick' in W. B. Yeats' poem 'Sailing to Byzantium', a metaphor for a spiritual journey, and George Eliot playfully asks in *The Mill on the Floss* why 'we can so seldom declare what a thing is, except by saying it is something else'. Metaphors are central to human thinking and communication. Contrary to the notion that metaphor is of some peripheral linguistic interest, metaphor is in fact pervasive in everyday life. Metaphor means the understanding, experience or communication of one kind of thing in terms of another.

It is difficult to get through a working day interacting with patients and co-workers without using a string of metaphors. I recently attempted to document the metaphors encountered in a single day but became fatigued, unable to keep up with the stream of examples in the first few consultations at the outpatient clinic. My metaphoric working day began with commentaries on the weather ('brass monkeys' and 'bucketing down'). I was forced to agree that it was, indeed, 'raining cats and dogs'. One patient declared that she was about to 'crack up' with this latest relapse of her arthritis, and described it as 'the straw that broke the camel's back', and which might force her to 'throw in the towel.' Another had been doing well in remission until 'the wheels came off', whereas a lady who was coping with difficult circumstances at home felt like she was 'walking on eggshells' trying to keep the peace within her stressed-out family, some of whom were 'over the top'. Then, there was a jolly man who liked to describe his wife affectionately as 'the ball and chain' and asked if 'the jury is still out' on the cause of his condition or if the plan is 'still up in the air'. Later, when a colleague called and asked if he could present a difficult case and seek my opinion, I responded affirmatively: 'Shoot.'

Medicine is steeped in metaphorical descriptions. The value of metaphors in medicine is that they create opportunity for a common language shared by patients and doctors. They help make sense of complexity and enable patients to conceptualise their problems. Metaphors, particularly those devised in the words of the patient, give a measure of control, a way of coping with the burden of illness. Down the centuries, patients have found it helpful to give an identity to their burden. Winston Churchill wasn't the first to transmute his depression into the *black dog* always in the background, in his lap and following him around.

Research has shown that metaphors facilitate communication between doctors and patients. However, like other forms of language, metaphors have limitations. Many become overworked or jaded clichés. At worst, they may stigmatise patients or unnecessarily introduce a sense of shame. For example, when doctors adopt the military metaphor for *the battle* against cancer, they may unwittingly make a patient feel a failure and experience a sense of shame, if they do not respond satisfactorily to treatment. Those who cannot tolerate side-effects of chemotherapy and opt for palliation do not need the added burden of feeling like a *quitter*. The military metaphor requires patients to be *tough,* implying that those who are *weak* may *lose* the battle. The oncologist in Edson's story informs Vivian that she has an *insidious* cancer and its treatment has *pernicious* side-effects. He tells her: 'The most important thing is for you to take the full dose of chemotherapy . . . you must be very tough. . . . Do you think you can be very tough?' Vivian, who has always been demanding in her own career, feels obliged to accept the challenge: 'Never one to turn from a challenge', she thinks to herself, as she becomes captive of the military metaphor.

Metaphors may be ambiguous, confusing and misinterpreted. Consider the patient struggling to get through a course of chemotherapy when told that 'It's all downhill from here.' Intended as encouragement, with the implication that freewheeling downward will be easier, the alternative interpretation of the metaphor is that if it is good when 'things are looking up', it must be bad if they are looking down. Other metaphors are distasteful. For example, primary care doctors are often relegated to the level of *gatekeepers* for an overcrowded hospital system, and elderly patients with nowhere to go after discharge from hospital are referred to as *bed-blockers.*

Then there are the horrible metaphors that unnecessarily add to a patient's distress. The *widow-maker* or the less familiar *widow's block* is metaphor for a narrowing of the left anterior descending coronary artery because of the high risk of a fatal heart attack. In a short story by Roddy Doyle published in the *New Yorker,* a cardiologist tells a man he has such a lesion, and casually mentions its metaphoric name. He is given tablets and lots of leaflets to read, but his thoughts are dominated by the metaphor. He can't even remember the cardiologist's face. He reflects on his past, his children, on the weather, but returns to his widow's block. How will he tell his wife she is going to be a widow.

WHO'S AFRAID OF SUSAN SONTAG?

Writing from her experience with breast cancer, and that of her father with tuberculosis, the American writer Susan Sontag railed against the abuse of metaphors in descriptions of illness. In her landmark polemic, she drew extensively on references in nineteenth- and twentieth-century literature to expose numerous myths and harmful stereotypes regarding cancer and tuberculosis. Many of the fallacies addressed by Sontag arose from ignorance about disease, particularly its causation. Later, she extended her study to AIDS (*Illness as Metaphor & AIDS and Its Metaphors*). For Sontag, disease 'could be considered as much a part of nature as is health'. She insisted that 'nothing is more punitive than to give a disease a meaning – that meaning invariably a moralistic one'. Sontag has been criticised for her polemical style. Despite her entreaty to avoid metaphors for describing illness, she begins her book with metaphors: 'Illness is the night-side of life, a more onerous citizenship. Everyone who is born holds dual citizenship, in the kingdom of the well and in the kingdom of the sick. Although we all prefer to use only the good passport, sooner or later each of us is obliged, at least for a spell, to identify ourselves as citizens of that other place.'

However, her important contribution was to challenge doctors and society to think about how language may distort our thinking about disease, and the potential adverse effects of language on patients. Disease should be itself, not be explained with metaphors which, in Sontag's view, distort or dilute the truth, or worse, may confer guilt, stereotype, shame, stigma or fear. According to Sontag, 'The most truthful way of regarding illness – and the healthiest way of being ill – is one most purified of, most resistant to metaphors.' But patients need to make sense of their illness, and need metaphors as a means of understanding, and as a coping strategy. Anatole Broyard noted that while Sontag dealt mainly with negative metaphors, positive metaphors may have healing power. In his whimsical series of essays on his own illness, and on life and death, Broyard wrote that 'Metaphors may be as necessary to illness as they are to literature, as comforting to the patient as his own bathrobe and slippers. At the very least, they are a relief from medical terminology.' He concluded that 'Perhaps only metaphor can express the bafflement, the panic combined with beatitude of the threatened person.'

THE PERSONAL METAPHOR

Patients should have ownership of their metaphors, just as they are entitled to their own opinions, if not their own facts. In the same way that patients make decisions about their treatment options, they likewise 'deserve to be the keepers of the lens through which they view their illness', according to Dr Dhruv Khullar. Not all metaphors are equal or effective for communicating complex issues. Whether the patient sees their dilemma as a battle, a journey, a marathon or a sprint, a rollercoaster or a chess match, or none of the above, will be determined by their need to personalise and explain their illness in a way that makes sense for them, and makes it easier to cope with. This will be influenced by prior experiences, education, values, culture and preferences.

One of my favourite pieces of sculpture open to the public stands in the foyer of the Cork University Hospital in Ireland. It is a steel sculpture entitled *Bandaged Heart* by the artist Cecily Brennan, who was inspired by lines from the poet Denis O'Driscoll ('Reality Check'):

> The heart should be cast in steel
> to spare it human feelings, wrapped
> in a bow of bandages, tourniquet to stem
> the flow from blood-corroded arteries.

Dedicated to all patients and families with hearts broken from loss and illness, *Bandaged Heart* can be taken as metaphor for the fragility of life and the universal need for support, including the gleaming stainless steel of medical instruments.

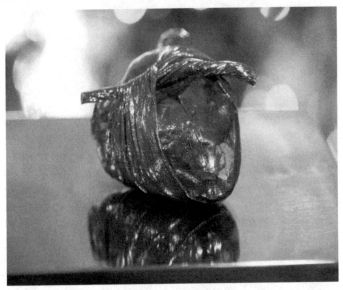

Subjectivity with metaphors in medicine and the significance of the personal metaphor was made clear to me a few years ago when my colleagues and I sponsored a symposium on medical humanities entitled *The Experience of Illness/Learning from the Arts,* which included an accompanying art exhibition on the same topic. The exhibition included the photographic work of Thomas Struth, including a series of photographs intended for patients and doctors in hospital. One of these images was a display of dandelions. Dandelions might be considered weeds by many people, but for others they are a thing of some beauty, a flower in the wrong place. One of the visitors to the exhibition, a well-known Irish radio and television celebrity, herself a survivor of breast cancer and a keen gardener, spent an inordinate amount of time with the dandelion image. For her, the dandelion was akin to a metastatic cancer cell in her body, and she regularly excised all dandelions from her garden lawn with great urgency. The image in our exhibition was unexpected for her but, with good humour, she adopted the view that it was a new opportunity for her to engage face-to-face with her feared bogey.

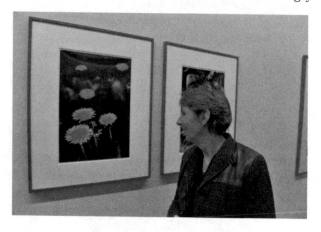

M&Ms scattered on the floor is how Lorrie Moore imagined cancer cells spreading, in her story of a mother coping with her son's malignant tumour, but the mother angrily rejects all other metaphors as inappropriate. 'It's a journey,' says the husband, but she is not interested in a journey. 'It's all very hard,' another mother offers. 'There's a lot of collateral beauty along the way.' But this is also unacceptable. 'A child is ill. No one is entitled to any collateral beauty,' she thinks. Finally, the husband asks: 'Don't you feel consoled, knowing we're all in the same boat, that we're all in this together?' No, the mother is not content to be numbered among other unfortunate families at the hospital: 'Who on earth would want to be in this boat? . . . This boat is a nightmare boat', and then she personalises the metaphor: 'Let's make our own way . . . not in this boat. Woman Overboard!'

Christopher Hitchens wrote about his response to the military metaphor for cancer when he was diagnosed with oesophageal cancer, likening the experience to 'confronting one of the most appealing clichés in our language'. 'People don't have cancer: they are reported to be battling cancer.' Well-wishers try to be positive: 'You can beat this', but sadly, obituaries are about 'cancer losers'. Although he found the imagery of a struggle to be somewhat appealing, his preference would have been different: 'I sometimes wish I were suffering in a good cause, or risking my life for the good of others, instead of just being a gravely endangered patient.' Hitchens is clear that when one is on the receiving end of an infusion of poisons, otherwise known as chemotherapy, 'the image of the ardent soldier or revolutionary is the very last one that will occur to you'. He concludes that he was not battling his tumour: 'it is the cancer that is making war on me'.

The battle-metaphor persists, despite the protestations of those who have experienced serious illness. Journalist John Diamond was emphatic that he was not writing about a battle or war against cancer when he wrote about his experience with throat cancer in newspaper columns and in his book *C Because Cowards Get Cancer Too*: 'I despise the set of warlike metaphors that so many apply to cancer,' he wrote. 'My antipathy to the language of battles and fights has nothing to do with pacifism, and everything to do with a hatred for the sort of morality which says that only those who fight hard against their cancer survive it, or deserve to survive it – the corollary being that those who lose the fight deserved to do so.' In recording his death, the *Irish Times* obituary began with the following line: 'The columnist and broadcaster John Diamond has died following a long battle with throat cancer.'

Doctors occasionally drift into metaphoric language by endowing cancer cells with intent, using words like *canny* and *smart* as they *learn to outwit* and *figure out* ways of beating immune defences. This is nonsense: cancer cells predictably acquire resistance because of the evolutionary emergence of mutant cells, not by some calculated design. Ascribing a cunning deviousness to cancer frightens patients and is biologically meaningless.

Dappled Things

'Glory be to God for dappled things' wrote the poet Gerard Manley Hopkins. Dappled is defined by the dictionary as 'marked with spots or patches, speckled and contrasting with the background'. People who become ill or disabled are like dappled things: they are different, and contrast with the background. There is nothing inherently stigmatising about any illness; stigma is created by the reaction of others to illness. This explains why news of a serious illness is often accompanied by an instinctive desire to conceal it. Serious illness is associated with heightened awareness, apprehension and even embarrassment in anticipation of how others will react. The illness-label represents a new kind of stigma, a transition to the other world of patients, distancing the sufferer from friends and others. Having a disability is similar.

Most patients want to avoid the awkwardness of changed relationships with friends and acquaintances. The English playwright

Alan Bennett recalled that when he was diagnosed with colon cancer, he felt a sense of shame and failure as he was paying his bill for the colonoscopy when the receptionist found it hard to look directly at him. Likewise, Christopher Hitchens wrote of the 'inevitable awkwardness in diplomatic relations between Tumourtown and its neighbours'. Robert McCrum has also recorded a sense of shame and embarrassment after his stroke: 'the majority of passers-by simply do not see . . . and/or threat you with a mixture of ruthless disdain and pitying arrogance.' Similarly, in the 2010 film *The King's Speech*, the reaction of others compounds the stigma of disability when a young prince and future king, handicapped by a severe stammer, is called to deliver a speech before a crowded football stadium. Struggling to enunciate syllables, his anguish intensifies on seeing the responses on the faces of those gathered to listen, who look downward, then away in disappointment and embarrassment.

Words and gestures adopt uncommon significance for the sick and disabled, who become acutely sensitive to subtle changes in the behaviour of others. The stigma of illness – the 'spoiled identity' of the sick, as Erving Goffman describes it – is an added, avoidable burden. Stigma depends on whether the ill are judged as being different because of their illness, or whether they are accepted for the entirety of their being. Accepting illness as part of the human condition is a difficult lesson to learn. Not until Robert McCrum had survived his devastating stroke did he realise that he had previously been indifferent and frightened of illness, but then concluded: 'Illness is OK. There's nothing wrong with infirmity. It's part of the way we are.'

Illness is also a mark of human individuality. To borrow again from Gerard Manley Hopkins, it has its own pied beauty: 'Whatever is fickle, freckled (who knows how?) . . . Praise him.'

STICKS AND STONES . . . AND STIGMA

How remarkable it is that illness and misfortune can be carried with dignity and forbearance, yet it is the insult of stigma that is the most hurtful for many. Ancient infectious diseases such as leprosy, tuberculosis and sexually transmitted disorders immediately come to mind when one thinks of stigma and illness. This receded as ignorance and fear in society were replaced by knowledge and enlightenment.

Today, one of the most stigmatised of human conditions is poverty and the illnesses linked with poverty. Illiterate peasants in Ireland who experienced unspeakable abuses under the oppression of a foreign imperial power during the seventeenth and eighteenth centuries, had no knowledge of literature but clung to the following poetic lines:

Ní h-í an bhoichtineacht is measa liom, Ná bheith síos go deó,
Ach an tarcuisne a leanann í, Ná leighisfeadh no leóin
['Tis not the poverty I most detest, Nor being down for ever,
But the insult that follows it, Which no leaches can cure][2]

There can be little doubt that stigma and prejudice continue to follow the underclass. 'How much worse do we sometimes handle those who are less well informed and articulate?' This was the chastening question posed by Tessa Richards in an editorial in the *British Medical Journal* on patient-doctor miscommunications. Most doctors and health service officials who deal with pleas for assistance or complaints will concede that inarticulate and semi-literate communications are unlikely to be treated in the same way as those which are grammatically correct. Theodore Dalrymple (aka essayist and clinician Dr Anthony Daniels) believes that the linguistic and educational disadvantages of the underclass 'transform a class into a caste'. This is also addressed in George Bernard Shaw's *Pygmalion,* a comedy about class and language, in which language sets Liza free, gives her independence and changes how she is treated.

The soft bigotry and low expectations with which the health service often greets the poor and disadvantaged is compounded by the language used to describe their problems. This is particularly evident with disorders of substance use. Stigmatising language like *drug abuser, addict, user, abuser, junkie, crack-head* and *drunk* should be replaced with non-stigmatising terms like *person with a substance-use disorder.* Similarly, patients who are in recovery deserve respectful language, such as *abstinent* rather than loaded terms like *clean* or no longer *dirty.*

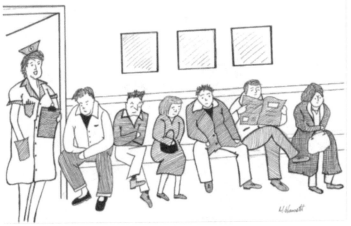

'Who's here for the drug abusers' clinic?'

Of course, language alone is neither the only difficulty experienced by these patients, nor the solution to better care. Understanding and greater medical expertise require better education and training of clinicians in the care of those with substance-use disorder. Meanwhile, unwitting or pejorative language among clinicians creates prejudice. Studies have shown that clinicians were more likely to take a punitive attitude when a patient was described as a 'substance abuser' rather than 'a person with a substance-use disorder', and were less likely to believe that the patient deserved treatment. More disturbingly, the stigmatising language of addiction isolates patients and is an important reason why those in need of help do not seek it.

STIGMA STORIES FROM SICK DOCTORS

When doctors get sick, they frequently speak of the comfort of knowing that friends and colleagues care, but this care is often lacking. Doctors who have written of their illnesses highlight the isolation, soft bigotry and discrimination that may be experienced when news of their illness becomes known to colleagues. Dr David Rabin was the senior endocrinologist at a major teaching hospital when he developed motor neurone disease. Relationships with colleagues that were once close, deteriorated after he was diagnosed. Few called or visited. 'Why this deafening silence?' he asked. Although the illness was incurable, Rabin asserted that 'There are so many ways colleagues can help'. The most chilling part of his story is the day he fell at work. As he lay on the ground, a fellow physician ignored him, and hurried past with eyes quickly averted, pretending not to notice.

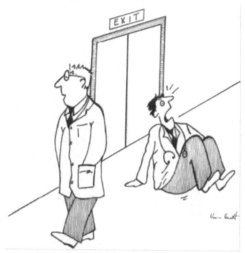

There are countless untold stories of the stigma of physical illness, but the difficulty for those with a mental health disorder is even more hidden. Dr Adam Hill, a paediatric palliative care physician, wrote an open account of his experience with the stigma of depression, suicidal ideation and alcoholism in the *New England Journal of Medicine*. Like many others, he had suffered in silence from what he describes as an 'epidemic of neglect' of physicians' mental health. His is a story of recovery, but also a series of lessons learned. One of these is the irony of a medical profession that has fought to change the stereotyping and shaming of patients with mental health issues, but is itself blind and neglectful of mental health stigma attached to its members with the same problems. When Dr Hill disclosed his history of mental health treatment upon applying for a licence to work in a new State, he was required to write a public letter outlining his treatment, which he described as 'an archaic practice of public shaming'. It seemed that it was not enough to be ashamed of the condition: seeking help for it was also a sign of weakness. However, disclosure for Dr Hill meant that treatment and recovery could begin. For him, it is not solely a matter of physician welfare; it is also important for patient safety. Physicians fear the repercussions of revealing their vulnerability, but Hill's experience has been that 'the benefits of living authentically far outweigh the risks'.

SCIENCE AND STIGMA

Stigma, negativism and discrimination contribute to the miseries of mental illness. Since stigma is usually rooted in ignorance, advances in the scientific understanding of mental illness have generated hope for greater acceptance of the afflicted. In particular, it was anticipated that knowledge of the genetic and biochemical basis of these conditions would have a de-stigmatising effect. However, some experts now feel that while the acquisition of a biogenetic explanation may dissipate attributions of blame or flawed character, it may increase the 'us-and-them' separation. If the problem is thought to be one of *bad genes*, the patient's experience of illness may be accompanied by a sense of pessimism for a lasting cure and may taint unaffected family members (associative stigma) with new labels such as *carrier* or *at risk* (anticipatory stigma). Whether this is a real or imaginary concern is still unclear, but establishing the facts through research represents an opportunity to shape public opinion, and will help reduce the stigma associated with mental illness.

Sadly, as science advances and ancient stigmas recede, they are replaced with new stigma-labels. On entering hospital, innocent patients are swabbed, sampled and tested for undesirable bacteria that reside on the skin or in the body. One might be forgiven for thinking that there are two types of patient: the MRSA-positives and the MRSA-negatives. MRSA (methicillin-resistant *Staphylococcus aureus*) refers to whether bacteria which are resistant to certain antibiotics are present on the skin. MRSA-positives are a potential threat to themselves and to others. However, much more undesirable than MRSA is the CPE stigma (carriers of carbipenim-resistant enterococci), because CPE is more difficult to treat, and nigh on impossible to eradicate. As a form of antibiotic resistance, it is highly contagious and spreads quite easily to others. Carriers of CPE feel doubly insulted: not only have they received this burden from an overcrowded healthcare system, but, having acquired CPE, they are treated by the same system as something 'dirty', they are labelled and isolated, and frequently their treatment needs are delayed or cancelled.

Tell It Slant

Emily Dickinson's famous poem entreats us to 'tell all the truth but tell it slant': the truth, she warned, might be 'too bright for our infirm delight'. She advised that words of explanation should be kind and gradual, and should neither dazzle nor blind. The message was similar in Dr Lawrence Henderson's famous address to the Harvard Medical School Colloquium in 1934: 'Above all, remember that it is meaningless to speak of telling the truth, the whole truth, and nothing but the truth, to a patient. It is meaningless because it is impossible; a sheer impossibility.' Henderson was not, of course, recommending that a doctor lie or present a falsehood to a patient. Rather, he was reminding clinicians of the complexity of any diagnosis, and the uncertainty surrounding the outcome. Drawing on the example of a cancer diagnosis, he pointed to the fact that no two cancers are identical, and no two patients are identical, and that the prognosis is highly variable. In addition to the fallacy of telling nothing but the truth, Henderson pointed out that to tell the whole truth may violate an earlier, more fundamental tenet of medicine: *primum non nocere*. As much harm may be done by telling the truth as by lying.

In Dr Jay Katz's study of bioethics and communication between physicians and their patients, *The Silent World of Doctor and Patient*, he poses the following incisive question: 'Can hope and reassurance be offered to patients without resorting to deception and without inviting disappointment?' He argues that acknowledging the limitations of medicine and of physicians does not undermine the placebo effect; rather, it still leaves room for hope and faith. Acknowledging uncertainty in medicine shows the physician's honesty and also creates room for hope and faith. 'Honest presence' and caring or non-abandonment is the reassurance that patients often seek from their doctor, not a promise of the impossible. When a doctor finds it difficult to provide hope, he or she should at least not deny it. 'I'm on your side' and 'I will stick with you throughout this' is the honest assurance that provides comfort.

People are not statistics, and people beat the odds all the time. It is not what people die from that is of interest, but rather what they are capable of surviving with. The famous evolutionary biologist Stephen Jay Gould addressed this in an important essay with a pithy message: '*The median isn't the message.*' This was probably a play on Marshall McLuhan's injunction in 1964, 'the medium is the message', which referred to how the characteristics of the media influence how we interpret messages. Gould was diagnosed with an aggressive form of cancer, abdominal mesothelioma, and knew from the medical literature that the 'median mortality' for this kind of cancer was then about eight months. The median is the mid value when data are in numerical order, and is the statistic most often quoted when oncologists refer to survival from cancer. Doctors who have such discussions with patients should read Gould's essay, the central message of which is that patients and tumours exhibit much biological variation – something which is not captured by a single statistic. In most cases, one cannot predict whether a patient's survival will be above or below the median. In fact, Gould beat the odds and died twenty years later, from a different, unrelated form of cancer.

Finding the right words to relay complex information without being patronising is not easy. To borrow from the poet Philip Larkin, the doctor must be able to find 'words at once true and kind, or not untrue and not unkind'. The words should be thoughtful, and delivered slowly. Any hint of deception through euphemisms should be avoided. For example, the layperson may interpret the word *treatable* as *curable* but may not understand the word *tumour* to be *cancer* and may not appreciate that a *secondary* implies *spread* of cancer.

Time is needed, often in divided doses. One meeting is seldom enough. Regardless of how informed the patient may be, my policy has always been: *Come back later.* Patients do not require perfection in communication skills from their doctor; they need time, kindness and honest presence.

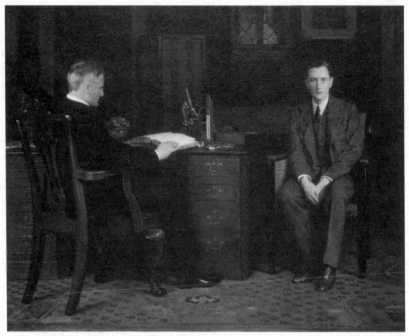

A physician telling a patient that he is going to die: the patient stares out at
the viewer. Colour photogravure after the Hon. John Collier, 1908.
Wellcome Collection. Attribution 4.0 International (CC BY 4.0)

8

⊷⊷⊷

Language Gaps and Words that Get in the Way

'When I use a word,' Humpty Dumpty said, in rather a scornful tone, 'it means just what I choose it to mean – neither more nor less.'
—Lewis Carroll, *Through the Looking Glass*

The All-clear – Hyper or Tense, or Both? – The 'Difficult' Patient – Pain Scales – Softer or Stronger Words – 'Second' or 'Secondary' Victims – The Tyranny of a Positive Attitude – End-of-life Language

Mr Humpty Dumpty's point is that words do not mean the same thing to everyone. They can be loaded with implications. They also change their meaning over time. 'Words are signals . . . they are not immortal', as shown by playwright Brian Friel in *Translations*. Medicine abounds with terms and syndromes that have outlived their usefulness and been retired from use. For example, *neurasthenia* (a form of mental and physical exhaustion thought to be due to depletion of nervous energy) was a popular diagnosis in the late nineteenth and early twentieth centuries. Several famous people, including Virginia Woolf, Florence Nightingale and Marcel Proust were thought to be afflicted with the condition, and neurasthenic characters were widely portrayed in popular Victorian novels. The word is no longer used; it was little more than a label to disguise ignorance, and was loaded with socio-cultural implications, often with a gender bias and stigma. The term may have allowed doctors to cater to patients' sensibilities, but it created confusion, and led to misguided treatments such as the 'rest cure', which was usually reserved for women. The 'rest cure', not only ineffective but hazardous, was famously portrayed in 'The Yellow Wallpaper', a short story by Charlotte Perkins Gilman, in which a wealthy woman goes crazy with the boredom of the 'rest cure' imposed on her by quacks.

In more recent times, doctors regularly prescribed a *tonic* for their patients, with the implicit intent of providing a boost for appetite, health and energy. The concept was shown to have no evidence-base, and tonics declined in popularity when their alcohol content was removed. Tonics are now consigned to the field of alternative medicine. Even the word *alternative* has become questionable in the context of medicine, since it may be contested that there is only a medicine that works, and anything that doesn't work is not medicine, alternative or otherwise. As I write this, I am also conscious that the word which describes my job, my role in society, is *academic*. I am a scholar, but to many people this word describes something of no importance: a fine detail of no practical relevance!

Here, we will explore further the limits of language for describing the experience of illness with examples of language-gaps and occasions where words get in the way, or even impede understanding.

THE ALL-CLEAR

In one of the episodes of the popular British television sitcom *Only Fools and Horses* written by John Sullivan, the two Trotter brothers, Derek 'Del Boy' and Rodney, each receive results of a medical test for a possible inherited disease. 'All clear! All clear! I got an all clear!' announces Rodney with great relief. Del anxiously opens his envelope, and with a horrified expression looks to his brother, barely raising his voice above a whisper: 'It says . . . It says, result of test . . . negative!' Rodney is stunned by this news but quickly recovers: 'Negative? Well, that means all clear, you plonker!' 'Does it?' says Del. 'I thought it was a medical term for curtains! Why don't they bloody well put all clear, then?' 'Who cares?' says Rodney, and the two brothers retire to the pub to celebrate.

Who cares indeed! No one would care if everyone understood a word in the same way. Malpractice lawsuits have arisen because of misinterpretation of a single word. *Positive* doesn't necessarily mean 'good', and *negative* doesn't always mean 'bad'. *Positive* only means that the laboratory found what the doctor was looking for, and *negative* means that the lab didn't find whatever was tested for. Consider the following example. A rare form of inherited immune deficiency is characterised by phagocytes (scavenger white cells) that cannot kill infectious organisms. This is called chronic granulomatous disease, and one of the tests used to diagnose it is the NBT (nitrobluetetrazollum) dye test.

The test depends on the reduction of NBT to a blue compound by white blood cells. The deeper the blue, the better the cell is. A positive test is normal; a negative test means that the reaction did not turn blue. The words *positive* and *negative* are inadequate for reporting the result of such a test, and predictably, this has led to delayed diagnoses of some patients with tragic consequences. For many diagnostic tests, there is no simple yes/no result; rather, the result requires interpretation in the light of the context, and the patient's complaints. There is no test for the all-clear, and all tests have risks, including false positives and false negatives.

HYPER OR TENSE, OR BOTH?

When ordinary words are given extraordinary meanings in medicine, misinterpretation is likely to follow. For example, when news broadcasters announce that those involved in a road traffic accident are now being treated for shock, it is assumed that they are being treated for psychological trauma, but in medical parlance shock is far more serious, and implies circulatory collapse.

Misunderstanding of medical labels using ordinary words was famously shown in a classic report by the American social anthropologist Dan Blumhagen in 1980. He interviewed patients attending a clinic for high blood pressure control. While the experts called this condition *hypertension*, most of the patients knew it as *hyper-tension* (too much tension). The transition from hypertension to hyper-tension was understandably linked to the belief by patients that it was caused by identifiable stress in their lives. They also thought that the excessive tension created physical symptoms. Such belief, in part, explains high rates of non-adherence to prescribed medications for high blood pressure. 'I know better than the doctor when I feel hyper-tense, and that's when I take the tablets, but now that I am calm, I can stop taking the drugs.'

THE 'DIFFICULT' PATIENT

At least one in every ten patient-clinician encounters is rated by the clinician involved as 'difficult'. Patients might put the figure higher. The asymmetries of the patient-doctor interaction discussed in the introductory chapter underpin some of the difficulties, but other contributory factors include doctors who are rushed and fatigued, or circumstances that are chaotic, such as a crowded emergency room.

For their part, patients cannot be blamed for being angry, frightened and stressed in the heat of crisis, but when patients are continually or repeatedly difficult with more than one caregiver, they become labelled: *difficult, problem, heartsink* or a *hateful* patient. This assigns culpability to the patient rather than the patient's illness, and seems to excuse the clinician from any responsibility. However, caregivers would do well to recall the injunction of clinician-poet Walter Carlos Williams: 'There's nothing like a difficult patient to show us ourselves.' Difficult encounters usually reflect the complexity of the illness-experience, and call for caregivers to exercise their expertise, compassion and understanding. Dr Bernard Lown had a better term, one which is kinder, insightful, and in the end, more useful: the *troubled* patient.

So that I May Feel Your Pain . . . on a Scale of 0 to 10

Pain is the commonest of all symptoms of which people complain. It is notoriously difficult to describe, yet a person in pain can speak of little else but pain. Joanna Bourke, a professor of history, describes how the language that people use to describe pain has changed through the ages, influenced by culture and religion. 'People in pain are often highly creative in expressing their suffering,' she says. Metaphors for pain have included fire, wind, colour, and weight. The language of pain, Bourke says, is not limited to words; it includes images, art, gestures, symbols, posture and performance. What about numbers?

'On a scale of 0 to 10, how would you rate your pain?' This is the usual question posed by doctors. The American essayist Eula Biss shows how incalculable the severity of pain is. As she sat in the hospital examination room, she wondered if it is possible to have a zero: no pain. What about emotional pain? And what about pleasurable pain, like sore muscles after exercise? The only thing that seems to be certain is that pain must be unpleasant, according to the pain experts.

A pain-scale needs fixed points, upper and lower. It also needs descriptors that can be shared. For example, the Beaufort scale used by mariners not only has numbers but also a term for the wind, the range of speed and a descriptor. Zero is not a real number for Biss – or at least not a number that can be added and subtracted or multiplied like other numbers. What about three? Three is nothing, according to Biss's father, who is a doctor: 'Three is a go home and take two aspirin.' It would be helpful if the doctors noted that on their scale, Biss thinks. There is also a problem with a five. This is 'the tyranny of the mean', which confounds scales from zero to ten, Biss's father says. Most patients tend to rate their pain as five unless it's excruciating. There is a preference to be average. After a year of chronic pain, Biss could no longer recall how it felt to have no pain. She laments that the pain-scale only measures intensity at one point in time, not its duration. A pain-scale, she believes, should have at least two dimensions. In addition, Biss points out that her pain is related to, but distinct from, her suffering. When she rated her pain at three, she had been sleepless for almost a week, and rated her suffering as a seven. The inescapable conclusion of Biss's account is that pain is unique, but it should also be shareable. The numeric scale, without fixed reference points and guiding descriptors, cannot adequately permit patients to share their experience of pain.

Guiding descriptors for pain have also been challenged by essayist Sinéad Gleeson, who has an extensive history of serious medical illnesses since childhood. The McGill Pain Index provides patients with a series of words, arranged in twenty groups of four, from which patients are asked to select those which best describe their pain. But these are the descriptors devised by doctors, not by the sufferers, argues Gleeson. This is a problem with almost all commonly used symptom questionnaires: they are devised by doctors, not patients. This has prompted the development of patient-reported outcomes (PROs) and Patient-Reported Outcome Measures (PROMs), the design of which is not easy, and should always include input from patients and consideration of those with low literacy.

How does one explain a specific pain to someone who has never experienced it? To reclaim the vocabulary of pain, Gleeson experimented with poetry, offering a personal poem from her own experience for each category of words listed in the McGill Pain Index, 'because pain cannot be reduced to one lexical bracket'. For example, she relates Hot-Burning-Scalding-Searing in the Index to her heartburn in pregnancy, but for Gleeson: 'It arrives like a stranger in town, an unfamiliar car cruising the street as mothers watch through curtains. This experience is commonplace for many, but new to me. . . . Words challenge the inferno, but turn to ash in my throat' and 'When I am not pregnant I resolve to eat jalapenos straight from the jar.'

Similarly, Anne Boyer considered developing pamphlets for patients with alternate vocabularies of pain based on the poems of Emily Dickinson. 'How does your pain feel today?' Response: It's a 584 (*It ceased to hurt me*) but yesterday it was a 650 (*Pain has an Element of Blank* and tomorrow I fear it may be a 1049 (*Pain has but one acquaintance and that is death*). It is said that references to pain occur in fifty of Dickinson's poems.

SOFTER OR STRONGER WORDS

Misnomers, ambiguities, paradoxes, inconsistencies, contradictions and imprecision abounds in medical jargon, as discussed in Chapter 2, but some terms have become problematic for other reasons. Euphemisms are used by politicians and bureaucrats to deceive, and everyone uses euphemisms to disguise or soften an unpleasant truth. In the memorable words of two great poets: 'Human kind cannot bear very much reality' (according to T. S. Eliot), but the trust between patients and their carers relies on the following advice: 'Tell all the truth but tell it slant' (Emily Dickinson).

The problem is that the disguise fades with time, and to remain soft, the words need to be refreshed continually. The evolution of euphemisms was part of a famous routine by the influential American stand-up comedian and social critic George Carlin. Criticising dehumanising euphemisms as the soft language that 'takes the life out of life', Carlin's insightful example was the extreme nervous stress experienced by, soldiers in battle. *Shell shock* was the description in World War I. Although misunderstood at the time, the term was simple, direct and onomatopoeic, sounding like the guns themselves. A generation later, in World War II, the term was softened to *battle fatigue*. This was then replaced by the phrase *operational exhaustion* and after the Vietnam war it became a form of *post-traumatic stress disorder* (PTSD). More syllables, less direct, less harsh, and according to Carlin: 'the pain is completely buried under jargon'. Adding pathos to humour, Carlin's concluding comment was arresting: 'I'll bet if they had still been calling it "shell shock", some of those Vietnam veterans might have got the attention they needed at the time.'

Strong language has its uses. Once was a time when the shock value of the term *battered baby syndrome* drew attention to an unpleasant truth in society that was poorly recognised and probably underdiagnosed. Similarly, *shaken baby syndrome* presents an image of human abuse of striking clarity. With time, these and similar terms have been transmuted into vague, all-encompassing terms like *non-accidental infant injury* and *non-accidental trauma*.

Time and context, along with improved understanding, are important forces for changing medical words. Words which have been uncontroversial and long established may outlive their usefulness, and become dangerous euphemisms. For example, the word *concussion* is generally considered to be a mild, transient alteration in mental alertness after a blow to the head. In many instances, this is an accurate description, but in the context of contact sports such as rugby and American football, where young athletes receive repeated blunt injuries, concussion is an insufficient descriptor. Athletes might receive better protection and attention if sports-related concussion were described as a form of preventable *brain injury*.

There are, of course, valid reasons for softening some medical words and phrases. Continual reform of disease definitions and terminology is desirable to reduce alarm, over-diagnosis and over-medicalisation of society (discussed in Chapter 9). For example, there is a strong case for renaming some forms of cancer that have a low risk of progression. Some low-risk tumours are correctly termed 'cancers' from a biological perspective but do not behave as cancer clinically, and do not need aggressive forms of management. Since language corrupts thinking, and may lead to unnecessary distress for a patient or unnecessary and excessive treatment, alternative terms have been proposed. The counter-argument has been that improved public education and understanding is the solution, and will avoid further confusion by the creation of new terms.

'SECOND' OR 'SECONDARY' VICTIMS OF MEDICAL ERROR

The term *second victim* was introduced in 2000 in an editorial in the *British Medical Journal* which called attention to clinicians who have made a mistake, and their need for emotional support.[1] At first glance, it seems reasonable to acknowledge that it is human to err, and conscientious doctors suffer when a patient is injured because of their mistake. Several authors followed, and soon it seemed as if *second victim* was the only one to suffer because of medical error, as reflected in the titles of supportive articles like 'Caring for Our Own' and 'Rescuing the Healer after Trauma'. While none would contest the importance of helping any carer who has made a mistake, the term *second victim* is flawed, and has been contested by families and patients harmed by medical errors. The label inadvertently diverts attention from patient safety, accountability, and the responsibilities of healthcare providers. Being labelled as a 'victim' may help the carer cope with shame and guilt, as it obscures responsibility and subtly implies that the error was unfortunate or random, because true victims are passive and lack agency. The primacy of the patient in all stories of medical error should be retained. Others may also need help, but they are secondary, not second, victims.

THE TYRANNY OF A POSITIVE ATTITUDE

Not everyone accepts the popular assumption that a positive attitude is an essential part of a patient's active management of their own illness, as proposed in many illness-memoirs of the triumphalist type. Barbara Ehrenreich has likened positive thinking in America to 'mass delusion' in her book *Smile or Die: How Positive Thinking Fooled America & the World*. Ehrenreich, who was afflicted with breast cancer, rails against subjecting patients to the popular notion that they must think positively, and rages against the pervasive 'pink sticky sentiment' in modern society. She notes that even the word 'victim' is discouraged, because of its aura of self-pity and passivity. Victimhood has been dismissed as being not politically correct (PC). This leaves no single noun to describe a woman undergoing treatment for breast cancer. Instead of a noun, verbs are used to metaphorically describe people bravely *battling* their illness or *fighting* their cancer.

When the treatment is over, the noun that is allowable is *survivor*. Sadly, according to Ehrenreich, the survivors' support club is welcoming if you're winning, but if you are losing your fight with cancer and have disseminated metastases (secondary tumours), you do not graduate to survivorship, and may find the club less welcoming. According to Ehrenreich, 'the failure to think positively can weigh on a cancer person like a second disease'. She was spared this 'additional burden' by her 'persistent anger'. Breast cancer, she protests, did not make her stronger or more spiritual. Rather, it gave her 'an agonising encounter with an ideological force in American culture that I had not been aware of before – one that encourages us to deny reality, submit cheerfully to misfortune, and blame only ourselves for our fate.'

Ehrenreich is not alone. Christina Middlebrook, a mother of three children whose breast cancer progressed despite the most aggressive medical and surgical therapy, rejects the notion that her cancer advanced because of her attitude. The healthy-minded approach, with its emphasis on positive thinking in popular books, only made her feel inadequate and guilty: 'I think dying is difficult enough without having to achieve a pleasant attitude.' Similarly, Kate Bowler, a young Canadian professor at Duke Divinity School, described the unhelpful life-lessons that people tried to teach her when she was diagnosed with advanced, or stage-four, colon cancer. In her book, *Everything Happens for a Reason and Other Lies I've Loved*, she is 'worn out by the tyranny of prescriptive joy' and rejects the your-attitude-determines-your-destiny advice. A more realistic wisdom from the popular *Perpetual Disappointments Diary* that is strangely satisfying advises that 'Everything happens for a terrifyingly random reason'.[2]

Prescriptive acceptance, dispatched with off-hand clichés like 'Things happen for a reason', 'It will make you stronger', 'God's will . . . works in strange ways', is another tyranny amplifying the suffering of patients in crisis. When Emilie Pine was distressed and needed to confide with someone about infertility after a missed miscarriage, 'Mother Nature' was invoked. In *Notes to Self,* she recalls, without self-pity, how she felt when 'let nature take its course' was the prescribed form of acceptance. Her response: 'no one thinks it's a good idea to let nature take its course when someone has cancer'.

END-OF-LIFE LANGUAGE

Everyone dies. Euphemisms may soften the fact for those left behind: 'She passed', 'We lost her', 'Deceased', 'Gone', but better words are needed by those who care for the dying. Like many clinicians, I have always been reluctant to write a DNR (Do not resuscitate) order on a patient's chart. This was never because I wanted to avoid making a decision or because of an ideological belief. The reason was the choice of words. Instead, I would write something like: 'Continue with all care and comfort for the patient but not in the event of a cardiac arrest'. I had the impression that the attitudes of the caring staff tended to change when they saw 'DNR' written. 'Oh, he or she is for DNR' they would say when handing over after a shift to their colleagues. The incoming team would nod, switch off, and focus elsewhere. In other words, it seemed as if 'DNR' was tantamount to 'Do nothing' or 'Withdraw all care'.

Changing the language from a negative to a positive statement can influence attitudes and actions, as shown when the term 'Allow natural death' (AND) was introduced in some American hospitals. The ethicist Daniel Sokol favours changing from *DNR* to *AND*, while acknowledging the imprecision of the acronym *AND*. However, this is surely one of the moments in a life when the gravity of the situation requires that caregivers resist using any acronym, and take the time to spell out respectfully and precisely an agreed plan.

The term 'the Good Death', used in medical circles, has been questioned by Dr Columba Quigley, who dedicated her early career to palliative medicine. 'Adding an adjective does not give us the control we think we might have, neither in relation to our own deaths nor to those we care for.' Death is unknown to us; adding an adjective does not make it more knowable. 'The Good Death' is acceptance of death as an outcome of care, an aspiration for control, but this is an illusion. Emily Dickinson's poem comes to mind: 'Because I could not stop for Death – He kindly stopped for me.' According to Quigley, 'Life, which includes dying, is a messy, chaotic and uncertain affair. We should not strive too hard to manage away the essence of that.'

Palliative care can, of course, offer much more than 'good death' care, but it has both an image problem and a language problem. Many patients who need it receive it too late because of previously held negative views. Negative phrases like *treatment withdrawal, futile treatment* and *ceiling of care* are distressful, undermine the concept of palliation, and give the impression that the patient will be denied the full potential of modern medicine. In contrast, language that is positive but not unrealistic, applied to what matters to the patient and his or her family, is comforting and hopeful. For example, treatment doesn't *stop* and is not *withdrawn*; rather, it is *re-directed* to *do everything* to ensure *comfort*. In a plea for better words for better deaths published in the *New England Journal of Medicine*, Dr Anna DeForest concluded: '"Withdrawal of care" would make an excellent name for a common medical mistake: turning away from the ongoing needs of dying patients and their families.'

9

⚜⚜⚜

Words that Turn People into Patients

'if there is a word for a particular thing we become convinced that such a thing exists'

—Richard Asher

The Dangers of Labels – What's Normal? – Medical Chic – The Medicine-seeking Animal – Maverick Priest – Non-diseases – Medically Unexplained Symptoms – The Most Neglected Word in Healthcare – Clever Words Create Vulnerable Patients – From Mislabels to Mistreatment – Different Words Change the Treatment – Wellness Language

When an enemy is given a name, it somehow seems less fearsome. Naming an illness may demystify worrisome symptoms; give a sense of control and a first step in defiance. However, labels have a dark side. They may confuse rather than clarify, offer little more than an illusion of understanding when none actually exists, and occasionally describe the non-existent; or, if wrongly applied, they may delay identification of the truth. In this chapter, we will explore how dangerous mislabels may be, the damage caused when normal is mistaken for disease, and how words can be used to turn people into patients and exploit the vulnerable.

A DISASTROUS LESSON ON THE DANGERS OF LABELS

When Leopold Bloom, the fictional everyman of James Joyce's *Ulysses*, meets a group of rowdy medical students, he wonders how they can become transformed from insensitive louts into pillars of society by the mere conferral of a doctorate: 'the mere acquisition of title should suffice to transform in a pinch of time these votaries of levity into exemplary practitioners of an art which most men anywise eminent have esteemed the noblest.' Unfortunately, the history of medicine includes several dangerous transitions, when the status of a normal process or variant is given a label. The creation of stigmatising disorders by identifying as disorder some normal variant of the human condition has often been born out of ignorance. Many of these misconceptions may have been harmless, but it is when misguided medical busybodies feel the urge to treat such fictions, that stigmatising, or more detrimental consequences, occurs. I recall as a child growing up in the late 1950s and 1960s that my left hand was tied behind my back at school to encourage (force) me to switch from being a leftie to a normal right-handed student. This practice was widespread in many countries but it appeared to have been pursued with particular relish in Ireland. Language may have contributed to this. Although derogatory terms for left-handedness are widespread (*sinister, gauche, southpaw*), there is a dedicated label for left-handed individuals in some languages such as Irish or Gaelic (*ciotóg*), whereas right-handers are . . . well, just normal!

Reflecting on the power of labels, the renowned paediatrician William A. Silverman recalled, when he was a medical student, hearing a city coroner announce that doctors who fail to screen infants for enlargement of the thymus gland should be prosecuted for malpractice. Long before the role of the thymus in immune defence was understood, it was thought that an enlarged thymus might be a cause of sudden unexplained death in children. The terms *status thymolymphaticus* and *thymic asthma* were introduced, and thousands of infants were 'treated' for the notional disorder with irradiation, to shrink the gland. This misguided practice continued into the 1950s. Decades later, it would emerge that the exposure to radiation in the children led to the development of cancers in other organs, including the thyroid and breast, in later life.

With the advent of specialisation, paediatric radiologists realised that the normal thymus gland creates a visible shadow on the chest X-ray of normal infants. Why had the earlier doctors failed to appreciate the range of normality for the size of the thymus gland? Dr Robert Sapolsky believes this was due to an over-reliance on post-mortem anatomic dissections from the poor and underprivileged. This led many to under-estimate the size of the normal thymus because the chronic stress and under-nutrition of poverty causes shrinkage of the thymus. In a sad commentary on the entire tragic saga, one of the pioneers of paediatric radiology, John Caffey, who was instrumental in refuting the thymus myth, said: 'Most mistakes I've seen were not because one didn't know some disease, but because [they] didn't know [they] were looking at normal.'[1]

A LITTLE BIT ABNORMAL AND ANOTHER BIT NORMAL?

What's normal? If humans have the right to be different, why do most people feel pressured to be either out of sight or within an acceptable range of size, appearance and ability? This is what Leslie Fiedler referred to as 'The Tyranny of the Normal'; in this article, he examines our historical ambivalence toward fellow humans who are perceived as deviant or outside currently acceptable norms, including the dangers of enforced normality when its definition falls into the hands of politicians and bureaucrats. Defining normal is far from straightforward. It perplexes philosophers and physicians, and means different things to different people.[2]

Normal can't be the same as healthy; it was 'normal' in Victorian times to have the stomach bug *Helicobacter pylori,* which was present in most of the adult population, but one wouldn't describe that as 'healthy'. Similarly, healthy is not the same as 'absence of disease', because many people who seem healthy have silent risk-factors for disease, and those who have chronic diseases, including cancer, commonly regard themselves as 'healthy'. Likewise, normal can't be the same as 'typical' or 'average', because most people in modern society are either obese or overweight, and that is not seen to be normal. If normal refers to a single trait, then most humans are a little bit normal and a little bit abnormal. Moreover, if normal is what we regard as the 'ideal' or 'desirable', then normal only describes a minority of the population. To pursue the 'ideal' or the 'desirable' is to pursue a moving target, because it varies with context and culture, and changes with time. Whatever its definition, normal should tolerate imperfection, acknowledge that variability is a biological advantage for the survival of any species, including *Homo sapiens,* and accept that illness and disease are a normal part of being human.

MEDICAL CHIC

A curious distortion of the desire to fit in with cultural norms is the acceptance of diagnoses which are à *la mode.* The gullibility of those who are impressed with fashionable diagnoses is portrayed in Axel Munthe's classic, whimsical memoir *The Story of San Michele.* Munthe was at once compassionate – treating peasants for free – and callous, in courting the rich and privileged, from whom he extracted a fortune in exchange for treatments of spurious and fancifully named disorders. In many instances, these patients were suffering with nothing more than unhappiness, boredom, anxiety or over-indulgence:

'Many were not ill at all, and might never have become so, had they not consulted me. Many imagined they were ill.'

His wealthy patients disliked being told the truth if they were over-eating:

'[Over-eating] was probably the most correct diagnosis I ever made in those days, but it met with no success. . . . Nobody liked it. What they liked was appendicitis . . . much in demand among better-class people on the lookout for a complaint.

However, when surgical removal of the appendix was recommended, 'a new complaint had to be discovered to meet the general demand'.

Almost sixty years after Munthe's memoir, Dr Michael O'Donnell's insider's observations on doctoring suggest that some doctor-patient arrangements include an agreed form of language for obscure illnesses that suits both parties. For the doctor, the patient's condition is not unduly challenging but requires frequent consultations, which happen to be quite lucrative. For the patient, the illness can be relied upon for an acceptable excuse to avoid undesirable social engagements and is one that engenders sympathy from friends and acquaintances. It is particularly reassuring to have an understanding and accessible physician. Loneliness is the problem, but that word is rarely acceptable and never used. As O'Donnell concedes, the distinction between treating the condition and exploiting it may be a fine line. Regardless, both parties in the arrangement usually settle on some form of acceptable terminology for the problem. This usually requires words that at once sound plausible and quasi-medical but lack precision. An extensive menu of terms to select from is usually available. These include: 'weak constitution', 'disturbed or sluggish metabolism', 'biochemical imbalance', 'hypersensitivity', 'food intolerance' and 'low blood pressure'. These conditions are curiously relapsing and remitting, and will have 'baffled' all the doctors who have been consulted previously. For treatment to be thorough and comprehensive, the condition needs to be carefully 'monitored', and will often require a vitamin injection with regular 'boosters', along with some form of 'tonic', in addition to the sensible advice for rest and perhaps a well-deserved vacation.

Borrowing from Shakespeare, Richard Asher wrote: 'A rose without a name may smell as sweet, but it has far less chance of being smelt.' Real or imaginary, a disorder is created once it is bestowed with a name, and a new group of patients, who have long been suffering in silence, come into existence. To address the unmet needs of these patients, there is commonly a band of therapists and natural healers peddling remedies, bluster and half-truths.

In some instances, the pharmaceutical industry has found it necessary to promote or invent a new disorder which is treatable with a drug for which the world hitherto had little need. The typical scenario involves a sponsored advertisement announcing the prevalence of Disease X, from which many are suffering in silence, but which could be controlled, if only the public were more aware of it. This public health campaign is usually accompanied by an advisory: 'You should see your doctor'. The impact is particularly impressive when a famous celebrity endorses the message. Spare a thought for the beleaguered doctor trying to manage an overbooked clinic, who is repeatedly asked if he or she is aware of Disease X, or will test for Disease Y, and what about Disease Z that a famous footballer says is treatable with testosterone-replacement injections!

THE MEDICINE-SEEKING ANIMAL

The worried-well in modern society represent easy targets for commercially driven outlets offering screening diagnostic tests and treatments for all the ailments of the Western World. One of the great paradoxes of medicine today is that we are healthier than ever, yet more anxious than ever about our health. Rising expectations and changing values have contributed to a perception of health as a continual state of youthful vigour capable of beating and cheating disease, decline and death. As the medical historian Roy Porter has noted, doctors have been turned into heroes because of their medical achievements, but still we feel equivocal about them. One of those heroes from an earlier era, William Osler, noted that 'the desire to take medicine is perhaps the greatest feature that distinguishes men from animals'. Unfortunately, consumers are not adequately equipped by our educational systems with a sound understanding of risk-versus-benefit analyses, or with the critical judgment skills needed to assess advertised health claims for drugs and other products.

Doctors have a responsibility to denounce the use of language designed to deceive. Health products peddled with slogans that have a scientific ring are particularly dangerous. The late Petr Skrabanek, doctor, scientist and polymath, pointed out that medical fashions have always come and gone, but the danger is greater than ever since the world became a global village with instantaneous dissemination of bogus messages. 'The financial exploitation of the worried-well and of the sick whom doctors cannot cure is no longer verbally denounced by the leaders of the profession; it is the order of the day.'[3]

LEGACY OF A MAVERICK PRIEST

When I was a medical student in Dublin in the 1970s, a Catholic priest achieved fame as a radical thinker and critic of institutions and professions in the modern world, including the medical profession. Most people were unaware that Ivan Illich was a priest, and viewed him as a kind of folk-hero beloved of political activists of the time. He appeared to be anti-authoritarian and controversial, but also deeply conservative. He appealed to populist opinion but was no common man. Like many intellectuals, he generated a mixed response of admiration and exasperation. Close analysis of Illich's writing reveals a mixture of truths, half-truths and absurdities. When he visited Dublin, the event was a sensation, packing the lecture halls with long-haired students and intellectuals. I still possess my beat-up copy of his book *Medical Nemesis,* which appeared in 1975. Its opening line – 'The medical establishment has become a major threat to health' – was revolutionary at the time, but insufficient to dissuade me from choosing a life in medicine. Illich was deeply critical of doctors, and argued that they probably did more harm than good.[4]

He was convinced that iatrogenesis (the causation of disease by doctors) was 'due to the doctor's control over the language of suffering', which he claimed 'is one of the bulwarks of professional privilege'. He attacked doctors by claiming they created diseases with technical language, and argued that much medical mystique could be dispelled with ordinary language: 'As soon as medical effectiveness is assessed in ordinary language, it immediately appears that most effective diagnosis and treatment does not go beyond the understanding that any layman can develop. The continued use of specialised language makes the deprofessionalisation of medicine taboo.'

While his prose could be obscure, he sprinkled it with provocative phrases that conveyed an unmistakable message: 'doctors' effectiveness – an illusion', 'defenceless patients', 'useless medical treatment' and 'doctor-inflicted injuries'.   Although Illich overstated the case against modern medicine, and was mistaken in his assumption that doctors actively seek to medicalise life and death in order to enhance their power and status, he correctly drew attention to the risk of overspending on healthcare, over-diagnosis, over-treatment, and the unchecked medicalisation of society. He correctly anticipated the abuse of language to create pseudo-diseases from normal variants.

Since Illich, a new generation of practitioners and commentators on health services has taken up the crusade against the excesses of health services and the overselling of sickness for profit. The concept of a 'medical-industrial complex' was coined by Barbara and John Ehrenreich and widely used in the 1970s; it was then popularised by Dr Arnold Relman, when he served as distinguished editor of the *New England Journal of Medicine*. The term 'disease-mongering' was coined by the medical writer Lynn Payer in 1992 to describe the activities of doctors and drug companies to expand the market for medical treatments by widening the boundaries of illness. In short, disease-mongering is the creation of more patients in order to sell more drugs. More recently, the campaign against selling sickness and over-diagnosis has been taken up by eminent scholars, clinician-scientists and journalists, including the Nobel laureate Dr Bernard Lown; former president of the Royal College of General Practitioners UK, Iona Heath; former editor of the *British Medical Journal*, Richard Smith; author and journalist Ben Goldacre; the late, great Petr Skrabanek; and investigative journalist Ray Moynihan.

When Is a Disease a Disease or a Non-disease?

Illness is what a patient experiences; it's what he or she consults a doctor with. 'Disease' is the name given to that illness by the doctor. However, much like the elusive nature of 'normal', the concept of 'disease' is neither straightforward nor static. Medical science continually identifies new diseases, most of which are caused by infectious, toxic or allergic agents, whereas other diseases are not really 'new' : they are just subdivisions of existing disorders, created by refinements in medical knowledge which retire old labels and replace them with more precisely defined entities.

In some instances, a disease is borne out of ignorance, or created for commercial exploitation. Part of the problem is due to the difficulty in defining normality and health. The World Health Organisation defines health as a state of 'complete physical, psychological and social well-being', but in a famous quip attributed to the late Imre Loeffler, this state arises only at the point of simultaneous orgasm – meaning that most of the time, most of us are unhealthy! Health and disease are usually ends of a spectrum, in which case one may have a little or a lot of them. Occasionally, they are discrete, as with an infection which you either have or do not have.

Richard Smith, the editor of the *British Medical Journal*, drew attention to 'the slipperiness of the notion of disease' and the 'increasing tendency to classify people's problems as diseases'. In 2002, he conducted a survey which identified hundreds of non-diseases. Non-disease was defined as 'a human process or problem that some have defined as a medical condition, but where people may have better outcomes if the problem or process was not defined in that way'. Most non-diseases are, of course, important to the patient, and suffering does not distinguish disease from non-disease: many with non-diseases may suffer as much or more than those with recognised diseases. However, non-diseases have one important characteristic: they are incurable with medical treatment. The non-diseases listed in Smith's *BMJ* survey included the patently normal (ageing), the seemingly trivial (boredom, unhappiness, cellulite and penis envy) and the more disturbing (loneliness). Whatever their remedy, kindness and time may help, but none of these conditions need drugs or medical meddling.

THE LANGUAGE OF MEDICALLY UNEXPLAINED SYMPTOMS

Medically unexplained symptoms differ from the non-diseases. Occasionally, they may be disabling, and more complex than most known diseases. However, all illnesses are real, even when lacking objective physical findings. While the term 'medically unexplained symptoms' may not have universal appeal, it is widely used, and has the advantage of pointing to the limits of medicine and the inadequacy of medical language. Medically unexplained symptoms are common, accounting for up to one in five consultations in primary care and a higher proportion at outpatient hospital clinics for specialities such as gynaecology, rheumatology, neurology and gastroenterology.

Doctors usually invoke one of two types of disease-concept to account for medically unexplained symptoms. First and most commonly, they may adopt a disease-label such as fibromyalgia, irritable bowel syndrome or chronic fatigue. The implication is that the label (disease) causes the symptoms, but the logic is circular: the symptoms represent the evidence of disease, which explains the symptoms. These disease-labels are also non-specific with overlapping symptoms, and many of the patients' symptoms affect multiple body systems. To compound matters, these conditions are often categorised in the minds of doctors as 'functional' – a word which is often hidden from patients, who could justifiably claim that a more appropriate descriptor would be 'dysfunctional'. An alternative disease-concept created by doctors for the medically unexplained symptoms is the notion of somatisation, in which the symptoms are attributed to some form of psychological or psychosocial problem that the patient denies or is yet to acknowledge.

Many patients find these disease-concepts unsatisfactory. Moreover, there is considerable overlap and variability in definitions when they are used by different doctors. The temptation for doctors is to resort to empiric treatments, which may add to the patient's burden and inflate the medicalisation of society, whereas patients want explanation and emotional support: they want their symptoms to make sense.

Medically unexplained symptoms represent a test of the strength of the doctor-patient relationship, which is often all that is required for treatment. An effective doctor-patient relationship is one of mutual trust, and will usually permit explicit language, whereby the doctor expresses words of *belief* that the symptoms are *real*, assurance that the symptoms will be taken seriously with an *open mind*, but with the concession that medical science often cannot adequately explain certain symptoms. The three most important words in education are 'I don't know'. They also acknowledge that ignorance and uncertainty are not only acceptable, but an essential component of medical expertise. Regardless of uncertainty, it is still possible to show confidence, optimism and reassurance: most medically unexplained symptoms usually have a good prognosis. Patients need to know this, and doctors need to tell them.

THE MOST NEGLECTED WORD IN HEALTHCARE

Uncertainty. Human existence is full of uncertainty, and medical science is immersed in it. Apart from death and taxes, uncertainty is one of the few certainties in life (although I like to add colonoscopy to the list). Failure to embrace and acknowledge uncertainty is one of the reasons for the medicalisation of society, and the over-treatment of patients with non-diseases and medically unexplained symptoms.

Medicine, according to medicine's grand old muse William Osler, may be considered as 'the science of uncertainty and the art of probability'. Lewis Thomas, author and physician-scientist, concluded that the major discovery from the past hundred years of biology has been the scale of our ignorance of nature. 'We are, at last, facing up to it. In earlier times, we either pretended to understand how things worked, or ignored the problem, or simply made up stories to fill the gaps'.

Despite remarkable forward-leaps in therapeutics, the exact effects of most drugs or surgical interventions on an individual are seldom fully known. Medical science has made it possible for clinicians to be clearer with their patients on the distinctions between what they know and what they do not know. Acknowledging uncertainty is a demonstration of expertise, not a sign of weakness. But uncertainty must not paralyse decision-making. As the eminent cardiologist Bernard Lown points out, the doctor must be an ombudsman for the patient, and this requires caring for the patient: 'only then can the physician somehow surmount the agony and absurdity of human decision'.

CLEVER WORDS CREATE VULNERABLE PATIENTS

Nowhere is the power of language more evident than in the naming of diseases. Labels are like infections that spread quickly and are difficult to erase. As William S. Burroughs put it: 'language is a virus'. Historic difficulties caused by mis-naming diseases were discussed earlier, in Chapter 2, and include the unnecessary stigmatising of people, and the creation of confusion. In 2015, the World Health Organisation found it necessary to issue a set of guidelines for naming new infectious diseases.[5] Long discouraged has been the use of eponyms, but now the WHO also discourages the use of terms that might promote panic, such as *fatal, epidemic* and *unknown*. However, the guidelines are for *new* diseases; reference to dubious disorders or spurious syndromes continues apace. This fosters the transition of the worried-well to new-patient status, vulnerable to exploitation for profit by those peddling unnecessary drugs and other remedies.

A characteristic common to man-made spurious syndromes is contagiousness: they spread rapidly by word of mouth and quickly become fashionable. Examples of some of the more popular conditions of the present day are listed in the table below. These conditions are steeped in controversy, but the reality of the symptoms borne by those given these labels is not in doubt.

Dubious diseases and spurious syndromes
Leaky-gut syndrome
Non-coeliac gluten sensitivity
Multiple chemical sensitivity
Adult testosterone deficiency syndrome
Acquired adult growth hormone deficiency
Female and male sexual dysfunction
Greater trochanteric pain syndrome
Adult attention deficit disorder
Social anxiety disorder (shyness)
Male pattern alopecia (baldness)
Premenstrual dysphoric syndrome

While doctors may use these terms loosely, knowing that they do not represent a definitive diagnosis, patients do not know this, and worry about something more serious. All illnesses are real, regardless of whether they are associated with physical findings, and although there are advantages and disadvantages to naming an illness, not every illness needs a name. What is important is that a doctor confirms that the illness is real, but that medical science lacks explanation for many such illnesses. Telling the patient the scientific truth is sufficient; a fabricated disease is unnecessary and potentially harmful.

There is, of course, nothing new about the creation of disorders for which a remedy can be sold. As a youngster I well recall advertisements claiming 'Guinness is good for you'; it was often recommended as a 'build-up'. The family doctor often prescribed 'a tonic' until it was revealed that the active ingredient in such concoctions was usually nothing more than alcohol. Later, vitamin preparations were peddled as 'stress tabs', the implicit benefit of which was for all of those feeling the stresses of life – which included almost everyone. However, when a product was linked in some way as a treatment or preventative for some worrisome ailment, the impact was greater.

Many will recall the slogan used to advertise Horlicks™, a nutritional drink: 'prevents night starvation'. Today, the word *Horlicks* is often substituted as slang for the less genteel *bollocks*. However, the product is still marketed, albeit without the bogus health claim. The striking use of the word 'starvation' was particularly memorable, along with the implied simplicity of the remedy for the problem if one were to buy the product. The clever slogan created a condition that does not exist. It was the creation of a man who was clever with words. In fact, it was the work of a minor but accomplished poet, Norman Cameron (1905-53), whose fascinating story has been told by Theordore Dalrymple (*Of Horlicks and Heroism*). Consumption of a sweet, fattening drink before bedtime was not an entirely harmless proposition, when one considers the risk of gastro-oesophageal reflux after one goes to bed with a full stomach.

When malodorous breath was transformed into a more serious disease called 'chronic halitosis', sales of an old product (Listerine™) rocketed. Listerine was named after Joseph Lister and invented as a surgical antiseptic in the nineteenth century. The highfalutin' name for bad breath, combined with advertising aimed at courting couples, turned Listerine into a highly profitable consumer product. The remarkable story of how 'Listerine did not make mouthwash as much as it made halitosis' is told in James B. Twitchell's book *Twenty Ads That Shook the World*.

FROM MISLABELS TO MISTREATMENT

When a disorder is poorly understood, there is a temptation to categorise or sub-classify it. Irritable bowel syndrome represents a good example. This is a real condition, but most patients dislike the label 'irritable bowel syndrome'. The bowel is neither irritable nor irritated, and the patient's symptoms are often not confined to the bowel. The only accurate part of the term may be the word 'syndrome', signifying a collection of chronic symptoms and signs. Difficulty naming this condition is reflected in the long list of disease-labels that have been used in the past to describe it. With some justification, it has been argued that the use of descriptive terms for poorly defined conditions should be abandoned, because it creates an illusion of understanding, when, in fact, none exists. To compound the confusion, irritable bowel syndrome is classified by leading academic gastroenterologists as one of a multitude of 'functional' bowel disorders. But what does that mean? Surely, functional should be *dysfunctional*?

All of this might sound like academic trivia, until one considers how patients may have been endangered by rigid adherence to sub-classifications of irritable bowel syndrome into so-called diarrhoea-predominant, constipation-predominant and mixed or alternating-type irritable bowel syndrome. Conveniently, the relative proportions of these notional sub-categories are estimated to fall neatly into thirds. This suits the pharmaceutical industry well, because it creates a market for the development of new drugs which target either diarrhoea or constipation – but are little more than expensive stoppers and starters! Unfortunately, none of these drugs addresses the underlying problem. Worse than that, the sub-categories of irritable bowel syndrome may be nothing more than misconceptions based on misused words. True constipation or diarrhoea are seldom confirmed by objective tests of stool volume and transit in patients labelled as having irritable bowel syndrome. Moreover, longitudinal studies show that patients may undergo transition between these apparent sub-types. Indeed, patients are often exasperated with these labels and declare that they can have constipation-predominant *and* diarrhoea-predominant irritable bowel syndrome all in the same day.

In February 2000, the US Food and Drug Administration granted the pharmaceutical company GlaxoWellcome a licence to market the use of Lotronex (alosetron) for the treatment of women with irritable bowel syndrome. Lotronex was an early example of a new class of antagonists of the type 3 serotonin receptor (5-HT$_3$). These compounds raise the visceral pain threshold and slow colonic transit. A randomised, placebo-controlled trial funded by the drug company and published in the *Lancet* in 2000 reported that alosetron 'was well tolerated and clinically effective in alleviating pain and bowel-related symptoms' in women with so-called diarrhoea-predominant or alternating bowel patterns of irritable bowel syndrome. Constipation occurred in 3 percent of the controls but in 30 percent of patients taking the alosetron. This was of sufficient severity that 10 percent of those taking the drug withdrew from the trial. However, the authors argued that this was not 'perceived as a negative consequence' of treatment. There was one case of ischaemic colitis but the authors of the study claimed it was a misdiagnosis.

Within six months of the launch of Lotronex on the market, reports of life-threatening side-effects, far worse than anything ever experienced by untreated patients with irritable bowel syndrome, were escalating. The two side-effects were severe constipation, sufficient in some cases to cause fecal impaction with obstruction, and ischaemic colitis. Untreated irritable bowel syndrome is a troublesome condition but is never life-threatening; yet, several patients treated with Lotronex died. The drug was voluntarily withdrawn from the market by GlaxoWellcome, although that was not the end of the story. Investigations would reveal that the risk to patients had been obfuscated. The integrity of the scientific assessment of the drug by the FDA was questioned; it seemed as if the FDA had become more a servant to industry than a safeguard for patients. The story has been recounted by the editor of the *Lancet* and by others. It reflects poorly on the pharmaceutical industry, the FDA's leadership, and the medical profession, and raises distinct regulatory and ethical questions.[6]

Missing from the accounts is an analysis of risk posed by the false premise that irritable bowel syndrome can be neatly sub-classified or sub-labelled into distinct entities based on symptoms. Although the authors of the major trial published by the *Lancet* conceded that 'no objective criteria exist for subgrouping' of patients, they specifically excluded women with constipation-predominant irritable bowel syndrome because the drug was expected to slow colonic transit. But how could they be sure that clinicians would accurately distinguish the correct sub-types, particularly if they didn't exist. Their study involved 119 sites in the United States: with so many doctors involved, it was almost guaranteed that the assessment of patients' symptoms would not be uniform. Moreover, the lack of uniformity was certain to be worse outside the rigorous setting of a controlled trial, when the drug was released to the wider world. Lack of precision and inattention to detail endangers patients, but particularly in the case of a potentially dangerous drug like Lotronex. The problem with sub-labelling irritable bowel syndrome is compounded by imprecise language. For example, patients with irritable bowel syndrome frequently experience a *sense of incomplete evacuation of stool* which leads to straining at stool, and which is commonly misinterpreted as constipation. The same symptom may also be erroneously interpreted as diarrhoea, because it causes the patient to make frequent trips to the bathroom. The distinction is important because it determines the type of treatment that is appropriate.

DIFFERENT WORDS FOR THE SAME CONDITION CHANGE THE TREATMENT

The over-medicalisation of society, which accounts for some of the escalating cost of healthcare, has deep roots, including the pursuit of perfection, with unrealistic expectations of what medicine can do, the misuse of some forms of screening, guidelines for treating almost every ailment, fear of litigation, direct-to-consumer advertising, greedy drug companies, and medical busybodies. But these are not the only drivers of excess; the words used to describe medical conditions influence doctors and patients. How much does the selection of a conservative or an aggressive treatment depend on the words used to describe the condition under treatment?

The influence of different terminologies on treatments was tested by a group of Australian investigators and published in the *British Medical Journal* in 2017.[7] They conducted a systematic review of published studies that compared two or more terminologies to describe the same condition, and measured the effect on treatment choices. Common conditions were assessed, and included low-risk ductal carcinoma in situ, reflux dyspepsia, conjunctivitis, polycystic ovary syndrome and bone fracture. The results showed that when a more medicalised or precise term was used for a condition, it was perceived as being more severe, and was associated with a greater sense of anxiety, and a preference for aggressive or invasive management. Patients have a lower sense of control over their symptoms when they are described in medicalised terms. Paying more attention to the language used to describe illness is likely to be most important when the risk of progression is low, and may help offset the assumption that immediate or aggressive treatments are always needed.

Most people will have either experienced conjunctivitis or seen someone else with it. Curiously, when the term 'pink-eye' is used, it is perceived as being more worrisome, more contagious, and in need of antibiotics than when described as an 'eye infection'. The reason for the difference in perception is unclear, but such preferences need greater attention and research. Another example is the term 'polycystic ovary syndrome', or 'PCOS', which causes greater anxiety and may be linked with lower levels of self-esteem by patients than when a less precise terms such as 'hormonal imbalance' is used.

Elsewhere in this book, the case has been made for greater precision with language. However, this needs to be measured, particularly in the case of low-risk conditions, to protect patients from unnecessary drug escalation and anxiety. Clinicians can support their patients' sense of control, and minimise the desire for tests and treatments, by choosing their words wisely.

WELLNESS LANGUAGE

Just when the world became saturated with selling sickness remedies for people transformed into patients by quacks and quirks of language, along came a new opportunity for charlatans and celebrities: selling wellness. In 1979, when the popular American TV news show *60 Minutes* featured an item on health, the host Dan Rather referred to 'wellness' as 'a word you don't hear every day'. Today, wellness is commonplace: wellness gurus, wellness programs and wellness tourism, all selling products and advice on how to live a wellness lifestyle. Some of the zealots of wellness peddle a deep suspicion of doctors, with an intolerance of the scientific method akin to that of a conspiracy theorist.

Once was a time when people had lives, not lifestyles, and their lives were consumed with the struggle for existence and supporting their families. Choice and control over one's life was a rare luxury. Today, there are lifestyles to choose from. The language of wellness sets perfection as the goal in life. We, too, can look like the celebrity! Perfect body and perfect looks, with no accommodation for illness, infirmity or disability. The wellness language cannot concede that illness, as well as health and wellness, is an intrinsic part of human life. Indeed, those of us who are well are probably more truthfully described as 'not yet ill'.

Claiming to be inspired by the WHO definition of health (not merely the absence of disease or infirmity but a state of complete physical, mental and social well-being), there is a dark side to the wellness business: the exploitation of the worried-well by using the language of fear. Danger-signs for consumers to be particularly wary of include extreme diets, elimination diets, celebrity endorsements and opportunities that are exclusive to the seller. True health and wellness lifestyles are free, and nothing can be bought that is likely to make us look like the celebrity.

The language used by the wellness industry is more akin to that of marketing than science. Vague pseudo-scientific terms like eliminating *toxins*, *detox*, *cleansing*, *boosting* the immune system, *chemical imbalance* and *de-stressing* are seldom supported by evidence, and usually have no basis in biology. When it comes to celebrity-endorsed diets, pat formulae and facile answers are the stock-in-trade. Scary messages sell (carbohydrates and fats are bad, but sugar is the real killer), whereas common sense and nuance regarding quantity and diversity of food seldom feature.

10

≼ᔕ≼ᔕ≼ᔕ

The Weight of a Word
Caring, Dignity and Empathy

'You should say what you mean,' said the March Hare to Alice.
'I do,' Alice hastily replied; 'at least I mean what I say – that's the same thing, you know.'
'Not the same thing a bit!' said the Hatter. 'Why, you might just as well say that "I see what I eat" is the same thing as "I eat what I see"!'
—Lewis Carroll, *Alice in Wonderland*

Contrary to what the March Hare would like to believe, words frequently don't express precisely what we wish to say. Insufficient vocabulary is not always the problem. When James Joyce was asked if there were enough words for him in the English language, he replied: 'Yes. There are enough, but they aren't the right ones. . . . I'd like a language which is above all languages, a language to which all will do service.'[1] When it comes to illness, honest words that are free of ambiguity are elusive. It is not easy to find words which can be shared by patients and doctors, and which are of equal importance to both. Some words might seem to be secure, established and bulletproof because of their common usage. Cherished words like *caring, dignity* and *empathy* appear to enjoy universal acceptance and consensus as to what they mean, but close scrutiny reveals surprising controversy.

THE PROFESSOR AND THE PLAYWRIGHT ON WHAT IT MEANS TO CARE[2]

Caring is a simple concept, cherished by professionals, but as a lived experience, it is more complex. Whether voluntary or professional, personal or public, caring means commitment. For some, it is another word for coping. It is a word for all of us, not just for doctoring and nursing. Sadly, 'caring' is a word which is often absent from political and economic debate.

Two great thinkers, both scholars of the human condition, have considered caring from different perspectives, both heartfelt and honest. One, a Harvard professor of psychiatry and anthropology, Dr Arthur Kleinman, writes from years of clinical experience and research; the other, British playwright Alan Bennett, addresses the topic in memoir and theatre.

Kleinman laments the declining status of caring as the great failure of modern healthcare. Caring has become a paradox. Whereas medical schools passionately uphold the concept of caregiving as 'core to health professionals' motivations and identity', they invest little in the way of time or resources to it, favouring technical competence, skills and knowledge. Doctors have become distanced from patients. The same seems to be happening with nurse-training.

Alan Bennett has written about kings and queens, but mainly about ordinary events happening to ordinary people, and how people care for each other. Although an admirer of the British National Health Service, Bennett has a deep distrust of caring. His views on caring are coloured by memory of his mother's illness; these views feature in works of his, such as *A Life Like Other People's* and *Untold Stories.* He also steered a diatribe on caring into his play *The Lady in the Van,* which deals with his interaction with an eccentric woman living alone in a van in his garden. His most recent play, *Allelujah!,* is set in a hospital ward dedicated to care of the elderly, and was called *Past Caring* pre-production.

For Bennett, caring is coping: 'Being landed with, being stuck with, having no choice about.' As a young man, he witnessed his mother's recurring bouts of mental illness, with which his 'Dad was left to cope. Or to care, as the phrase is nowadays. Dad was the carer.' He and his brother 'cared, of course' but 'still had lives to lead: Dad was retired – he had all the time in the world to care.'[3] Conscientiousness and devotion to duty is what killed him, according to Bennett. Familial madness is how the playwright describes his mother's illness. His devoted father preferred euphemisms ('This business with your Mam' and 'This flaming carry-on'). The doctors just called it 'depression' because they did not know her. When his mother was hospitalised, Bennett longed to take her away from 'this yelling hell-hole'. His father, who loved her dearly, travelled there every day, firm in the conviction that he must be there for her when she regained her sanity, because no one, including the doctors and nurses, knew her as he did. Years later, Bennett returned to devotional care in his play *The Madness of George III.* Like the playwright's parents, Queen Charlotte remains forever devoted to her husband: 'It is the same with all the doctors . . . none of them knows him . . . . So how can they restore him to his proper self, not knowing what that self is.'

In the screenplay for *The Lady in the Van*, Bennett splits his own character into dual *dramatis personae,* one coping with a difficult, irascible, non-paying guest, the other curiously observing the interaction as the ungrateful tenant ages and becomes frail. The playwright stridently professes his dislike for the word 'caring' when a social worker refers to him as 'the carer': 'Do not call me the carer. I am not the carer. I hate caring. I hate the thought. I hate the word. I do not care and I do not care for. I am here; she is there. There is no caring.' Coping *with* rather than caring *for*, is how he sees his relations with the demanding, ungrateful lady in the van. 'She is just something that's happening,' he remonstrated. Why he tolerated the situation, and for so long, is unclear. Was it a fascination with eccentricity, an author's desire for interesting material? Or perhaps it was guilt, a word seldom far from the word 'care', which also features in the play. Was it residual regret for his own inadequacy and impatience during his mother's illness?

The words used by Bennett for how his father was left to cope with his wife's illness, are not dissimilar to those of Professor Kleinman, who concedes that he only became a carer by necessity when his wife became ill: 'I learned to be a caregiver by doing it, because I had to do it; it was there to do.' Kleinman's wife, Joan, developed early-onset Alzheimer's disease, and his life was transformed by becoming her primary caregiver. 'We are caregivers because we practise caregiving.' It is thrust upon us, but according to Kleinman, it is the little things – the doing, the feeling, and yes, even the inadequacy – that make us caregivers.

Kleinman has come to view caregiving as a 'moral experience', an 'odyssey in becoming human', and an active 'presence'. Presence is a commitment to being there; it is an act of participation in the illness-story of another, and it is recognisable when it is absent. This aligns with Bennett's account of his father's insistence on being continually present for his wife, and perhaps with the playwright's guilt because of his own absence.

Whereas the professor uses profound, meditative language in his analysis of caring for a loved one, the playwright forthrightly attacks the language relating to caring for the elderly. For the professor, caregiving is 'to learn how to endure, the act of going on and giving what we have.' For the playwright, it is 'soldiering on: that was always how Dad used to put it and now I do the same.' Describing his own visits to his mother as a 'perfunctory duty', he was relieved when it was over. He is impatient with the 'blurred classifications' used in nursing homes for the elderly. Are they patients or inmates? Are they dying, or just incapable of living? Are the nurses really nurses? He winces at the childlike dialogue between carers and the elderly, likening it to bad acting. Contrary to what is implied in the word 'caring', it is seldom a 'gentle business', according to Bennett. Introducing *Lady in the Van*, he argues that when anyone says 'We have to do everything for them', it means 'We have to do one thing for them . . . clean them up.' He has used similar lines before and since, in short stories and in the play *Allelujah!*

Professor and playwright concur that caregiving is less about doctoring than many believe, and more about what it means to be human. Bennett recalls the doctor in charge of his mother's care as 'kindly and understanding, but as weary and defeated as someone out of Chekhov'. Reduced time spent with patients has diminished the caring role of clinicians, and in part, contributed to the modern pandemic of physician burnout. Almost a century ago, Dr Francis Peabody wrote that the secret of the care of the patient is in caring for the patient. From the testimony of Peabody's wife, he was aware that his comments on patient care would outlast any of his scientific contributions, but he was unlikely to have known that caring for the patient would also become the secret to physician welfare. Clinicians need more time *with* patients to care *for* patients. Moreover, by embracing the ordinary and by feeding their curiosity about patients and their stories, they can remain fresh and effective. Regardless of whether carers act in a professional or personal capacity, they need to be valued by society and supported in their endurance. Caregivers can benefit from their acts of kindness, but the regenerative power of caregiving needs to be nourished. Kindness and compassion are a limited source of human motivation, and should not be taken as granted.

Caring, of course, has a wider social sweep, beyond that of healthcare. Kleinman contends that caregiving should shape our political interaction with the rest of the world ('humankind's shared project'). If caregiving were a core value in society, global issues such as poverty, human trafficking, immigration, and famine relief might be handled differently by governments. This noble thinking accords with the Bennettian view of modern life in *Allelujah!,* where the common good is sacrificed for self-interest, and where heartless politicians preside over a contemporary society which has become insensitive to the predicament of migrants and to the care of the elderly.

With divergent minds and different perspectives, the professor and the playwright converge on what it means to care. For all its paradox and ambiguity, caring may be simple endurance – indistinguishable from coping – but it is core to what it means to be human. It transcends cultural boundaries. Caring for one another may be the difference between survival and the extinction of humanity.

DIGNITY, A USELESS CONCEPT?

'Dignity is a useless concept in bioethics', announced the bioethicist Ruth Macklin in 2003 in the *British Medical Journal*. She was not claiming that humans lack intrinsic dignity. Rather, she was questioning loose language and hollow rhetoric surrounding the word. In particular, she doubted whether dignity was anything more than a demand for respect for a person, and for an individual's autonomy. In full support of human autonomy and the rightfulness of respect for all humans, Macklin's stirring article was a caution against the unwitting use of words as superficial slogans – which, in the end, undermine their intended purpose. Her challenge provoked an academic storm, with one expert advocating at least five different forms of human dignity, but a coherent definition has not emerged from the philosophical fog.

The Harvard linguist Steven Pinker weighed in on Macklin's side. He points to three features which undermine popular concepts of dignity. Firstly, he points out that dignity is *relative*. Some people think that being hospitalised in a public ward rather than in a private room is beneath their dignity. Others seem to think that licking an ice-cream cone is undignified, whereas Pinker (and I too) have no problem with it. Secondly, dignity can be *substituted*; it is *exchangeable*. Modern medicine is 'a gauntlet of indignities', according to Pinker. Anyone who has had a rectal or pelvic examination, or a colonoscopy, will understand what he means, but we regularly trade our dignity for the results of such tests. Finally, Pinker argues that there are instances when dignity may be *harmful*. In support of this, he points to the ostentatious displays of the trappings of dignity by tyrants: medalled monsters in full regalia, demanding respect from their lofty pedestals as they review marching armies and weapons of mass destruction. He also points to the violence through the ages that has been inflicted in the name of dignity, on those who dissent from religious or political domination.

Of course, dignity is not devoid of value. It is really a matter of human perception, according to Pinker. The perception of dignity triggers respect for the dignified person. Whereas dignity is superficial, it is respect that ultimately counts for the person. This is how the concept of dignity applies to medicine, and how attention to the dignity of patients should be maintained if it does not compromise other aspects of care. In this sense, no one could disagree that the dignity of a patient is a standard for healthcare. History has shown that when this standard fades, or when the dignity of a person is diminished, a hardening of the heart may ensue: a callousness or desensitisation among the carers. Dignity also has value as a strategy for patients to use in defiance against illness and its humiliations. One thinks of the story told by Ashley Montagu of John Merrick, 'the Elephant Man', whose dignity stood in defiance of hideous disfigurement and deformities. Hidden stories throughout the ages feature people coping with illness and disability with great dignity.

Academic wrangling over the meaning of dignity continues. Reassuringly, most responses to Macklin's provocation have been impassioned, with a widespread desire to uphold the dignity of patients, regardless of how vague the term may be. The word has deep significance for patients and their loved ones. Like much of what we value, we know dignity best when it goes missing.

THE LEAST OF THESE IS EMPATHY

It is difficult to define what makes a good doctor. Easier it is to list what patients need from their doctor: competence, understanding, respect, time, compassion and kindness. Simple words: 'Now is a time for simplicity. Now is a time for, dare I say it, kindness' says an anguished Vivian Bearing, who is dying with ovarian cancer in Margaret Edson's play. She no longer seeks a cure, just 'the touch of human kindness'.

Why then does the philosopher Havi Carel write that empathy is the human emotion in greatest shortage in her celebrated book, *Illness: The Cry of the Flesh*? She feels that nowhere is this deficit more evident than in illness. But is she really calling for some compassion and understanding and more emotional engagement from her carers? Invoking the word 'empathy' is unnecessary: simpler words and concepts, like kindness and compassion, are more direct, understandable and sufficient. The word 'empathy' is relatively new in healthcare. It was rarely, if ever, used by great thinkers and practitioners of medicine, like William Osler and Francis Peabody, who wrote sensitively about the care of the patient.

Any word that continually needs definition, explanation and qualification should be treated with suspicion or discarded. In healthcare, the word 'empathy' has become clichéd, misused and abused. Superficial use of the term debases the concept.

I feel your pain. Sure you do! Would you like some more of it, then?

Empathy has also become, for some enthusiasts, a profitable commercial opportunity to sell empathy training. Since the elements of such training are already encompassed in good communication skills, the need to invoke empathy in healthcare is dubious. Several other considerations cast doubt on the concept of empathy in healthcare: it is unrealistic, unusual and occasionally undesirable.

True empathy is actually impossible in many clinical scenarios, such as a man caring for a woman in labour, an adult nursing a sick child, a woman physician treating a male with inflammation of the testicles (orchitis), or *cis*-males and females managing transgender-related illness. In such situations, kindness, compassion, understanding and competence more than suffice. Perhaps the same applies in all clinical circumstances.

Although doctors who have been ill may come close to the ideal of empathy by drawing on their own personal experience, and others may occasionally derive a sense of what it feels like to be sick from fictional accounts of illness, it is doubtful whether true empathy for all patients is achievable. Whereas disease is black, white and grey, the experience of illness is individual and unique, and coloured by context. No one can truly understand what an ill person is feeling. As Dr Solomon Papper said while he was being treated for cancer: 'Physicians and nurses, however much they strive to understand the total patient, may only comprehend something of his [or her] brain, intellect, and what his [or her] understanding of the disease is. It is more difficult to get into a patient's heart.' While in the depths of his own sadness, a young doctor said to him: 'I know just how you feel.' He found himself suddenly angry and said: 'The hell you do.' For this doctor/patient, empathy was just a metaphor, not a reality.

Objective physical responses to the suffering of others can be measured. These range from galvanic skin responses (sweaty palms and fast heart rate) to so-called mirror neurons or areas of the brain that light up on special brain-scans. Although often cited as biomarkers of empathy, they merely reflect human responses to the suffering of humans. Like other physical responses, they may be sensitised or de-sensitised. Jane Macnaughton is like most people: she experiences emotional distress on hearing the stories of patients, but this is not true empathy:

The sadness, or fear, or whatever feeling I have experienced is not sustained, and is so different from what the patient is feeling that it seems disrespectful to suggest that I somehow participate in his or her experience.

Macnaughton is co-director of the Centre for Medical Humanities in Durham, UK, and doubts whether it is possible for doctors to identify emotionally with their patients' illness in the truest sense. For this reason, she also believes that empathy should not be viewed as a skill or measured, as claimed by some medical schools.

According to Macnaughton, the doctor-patient relationship makes empathy impossible because of 'a mismatch of perspectives' – subjective for the patient and objective for the doctor. Of course, clinicians can identify with the physical aspects of a patient's experience, such as the feeling of pain, cold, heat or numbness, but a deeper appreciation of the patient's suffering is not possible, 'because the only access to my mind lies in what I say and how I look', as Macnaughton puts it. Looking and listening is not the same as understanding 'what I am feeling and thinking'. Therefore, she sounds the following warning:

> A doctor who responds to a patient's distress with 'I understand how you feel' is likely, therefore, to be both resented by the patient and self-deceiving.

I feel *for* you is not the same as I feel *with* you.

In an analysis of the limitations of the pain-scale used by many doctors, the essayist Eula Biss noted that her father, who is a doctor, declared that he had no pain when he broke his collarbone. While suspicious of his assessment of his own pain, the problem of pain, she wrote, is that 'I cannot feel my father's, and he cannot feel mine'. This, she believes, is the 'essential mercy of pain'. She also found comfort in the fact that no one can compare her pain with that of others, and for that reason it could not be proven to be insignificant.

Could empathy be undesirable in some circumstances? Doctors called upon to make decisions on hundreds of patients in a working week would be overwhelmed and incapacitated if they were to share in their patients' experiences of illness. Moreover, the ill often make poor judgements and need the assistance of clear-minded doctors, not doctors disabled with the same illness-feelings. Patients in despair following news of a serious diagnosis need reassurance, not more despair from their doctor. This argument is made by psychologist Paul Bloom in his book *Against Empathy: The Case for Rational Compassion.* While not rejecting the value of empathy outright, Bloom points out that other considerations, such as compassion, honesty, professionalism, calm competence and respect, trump empathy in medicine. He also identifies the important distinction between *understanding* how a patient feels and *feeling* how a patient feels:

> There is a world of difference . . . between understanding the misery of the person who is talking to you because you have felt misery in the past, even though you are now calm, and understanding the misery of the person who is talking to you because you are mirroring them and feeling their misery *right now*. The first, which doesn't involve empathy in any sense, just understanding, has all the advantages of the second and none of the costs.

In all human interactions, there is, of course, value in considering the perspective of a patient, a client, collaborator or opponent, and how they might be thinking. Understanding is central to negotiation and communication skills. Alan Alda, the famous actor and founder of the Center for Communicating Science at Stony Brook University, became interested in empathy, in part from a bad experience with a dentist, and in part because of his interest in communication skills and the importance of 'relating' to his fellow actors on stage. For Alda, empathy is central to good communication, and is the capacity to be aware of and relate to what is in the mind of another person. This is what actors call *relating* to one another. Elsewhere in this book, I have discussed the parallels between acting and the doctor-patient relationship, and Alda addresses how acting skills can inform and improve medical consultations. Good communication, says Alda, requires responsive listening and a willingness to be changed; that is, to hold an open curiosity in readiness to change one's opinion in response to the speaker. Bad communication is simply waiting to speak. In the course of his studies, Alda has refined his thinking on the process of relating to others. He has explored improvisation games to heighten awareness of what others are thinking and feeling (empathy), and found improvisation to be of assistance not only to actors, but also to scientists, medical students, and patients with autistic-spectrum disorders. There is much to admire about Alan Alda's approach and commitment, but awareness and understanding, which are commendable, are not the same as feeling the same feeling (empathy).

When doctors are criticised for lack of empathy, it is usually, in fact, for lack of compassion and kindness. In the past, trainee doctors were sensitised to the role of kindness and compassion by role-models. Today, a more formal approach is adopted by most medical schools with programmes in medical humanities, communication skills, and what is referred to by many as 'empathy skills'. However, the notion that effective doctoring can be reduced to an empathy index of checklists is simplistic. This has drawn the attention of several non-medical authors. In the opening essay of Leslie Jamison's 2014 *The Empathy Exams*, she describes her experience acting as a standardised patient for medical students and scoring them on their skills, and whether they used the correct words to get credit for 'voiced empathy for my situation/problem'.

She became sceptical about the formulaic notion of empathy, as the students adapted or gamed the system: they played the empathy game. While she reports coldness and lack of apparent sympathy with her concerns by some doctors, she also noted that others maintained their distance but were reassuring in their objectivity and calmness. Empathy, she concludes, 'is a kind of care but it's not the only kind of care, and it's not always enough. . . . I needed to look [at the doctor] and see the opposite of my fear, not its echo.' Alan Bennett addresses similar issues in his 2011 novella *The Greening of Mrs Donaldson*, in which a recently widowed woman finds a liberating lease of life when she takes a part-time job acting out illness-stories for medical students. However, Mrs Donaldson engages in a bit of her own gaming, with some enigmatic improvisation. She shows the importance of candour, sincerity and how doctors, if curious, can learn a lot from their patients. 'Here am I trying to teach counterfeit compassion,' says the senior medical tutor to Mrs Donaldson, 'and you're teaching them something else.'

In weighing the elements of effective doctoring, Dr Richard L. Landau of the University of Chicago explains: 'Effective physicians give patients sufficient time. . . . They will be sensitive, sympathetic, imperturbable, understanding, and occasionally empathetic, but by far the least employed of these traits will be empathy.'

11

✥✥✥

Language, Logic, Policy and Poor Public

Health Messages

'In my experience there is plenty of information in the world, but very little sense made of it'

—Eula Biss

If You Have Symptoms, It's Diagnosis Not Screening – Is Everything a Risk-factor for Something? – Misleading Misnomer – Obesity Distorted by Bad Language – Antibiotic Resistance – Changing the Narrative on Vaccination – Weary from Awareness

When Dr Samuel Johnson said that 'public affairs vex no man', he probably meant that we only become engaged with public matters that touch us personally, and regard other things in the world, if at all, with detachment.[1] This was perhaps true of public affairs in Johnson's eighteenth century, but in the twenty-first century public policy and public behaviour should concern everyone, because of their influence on personal health. In many respects, there is a convergence of public and personal health. Personal health is shaped by the wider social, economic and environmental context,[2] and as with personal thoughts, language influences logic, political decisions and public policy. However, in the same way that language-gaps between doctors and patients are a health-hazard, misuse of language also leads to flawed logic, and ineffective and damaging public health messages. The following examples of mixed messages and confused policy relate to the major public health challenges of our time.

IF YOU HAVE SYMPTOMS, IT'S DIAGNOSIS NOT SCREENING

If you have symptoms, a doctor may do a test to help explain the symptoms (diagnosis). The situation is very different when a doctor offers a test to a person who has no such complaints (screening). Politicians, even those responsible for health services, often misunderstand the distinction. Likewise, angry protests that patients might not have died, had they been 'screened', are often misplaced. Diagnostic tests prompted by a patient's symptoms have a different risk/benefit ratio, and are more likely to be conclusive than when a screening test is performed on someone with no symptoms. The distinction is important, not semantic.

Screening is for people who have not yet developed symptoms of disease; it is not about diagnosing people who are ill. The objective is to identify disease at an early stage, or to identify those who are at greatest risk of developing the disease. The benefit may seem obvious, but health screening is not a clear-cut issue. Some screening tests have many limitations. These include false negatives, which provide a false sense of security, and false positives, which may lead to unnecessary additional tests, anxiety, over-treatment and harm. Moreover, the false-positive rate rises as the prevalence of the disease being screened for falls. Even when screening picks up a disease earlier, the outcome is not necessarily better. This is because of *lead-time bias*. Lead-time is the interval between the detection of disease by screening and the point when diagnosis based on symptoms would have occurred without screening. In other words, finding the disease due to screening does not necessarily mean that the course of the disease can be altered, but lead-time bias makes it seem like survival is longer when the time of death is the same. This is an important factor in judging the value of a screening test.

IS EVERYTHING A RISK-FACTOR FOR SOMETHING?

Most doctors deal with individual patients one at a time, but epidemiologists and public health doctors study diseases within the population. Identifying risk factors or behaviours that predispose people to disease is a prominent part of the job of an epidemiologist. Some of the great historical detective stories of epidemiology include linking a water-borne transmissible agent with cholera, linking smoking with lung cancer, and identifying various environmental exposures with certain types of cancer. Indeed, much of what is known about the risk of heart disease and cancer has been generated by epidemiologists. Of course, epidemiologists have had some monumental failures: despite decades of research, they failed to identify that peptic ulcers and stomach cancer are caused by a transmissible infectious agent (eventually shown to be the bacterium *Helicobacter pylori*).

Epidemiology studies are also prone to misinterpretation because of widespread failure to distinguish between relative and absolute risks.

Relative risk is always expressed relative to something else, whereas *absolute risk* is expressed as a number out of 100 or 1000. Failure to make the distinction creates sensational news items and futile public health scares. For example, if a particular lifestyle behaviour increases the risk of a disease by 100 percent (two-fold increase) but the absolute is rare (say 1 in a million), then twice this (2 in a million) is still rare, and not worth worrying about. People who take two overseas holidays annually have an increased risk of death from an air-crash (twofold that of a person who only travels once annually). Since the absolute risk of an air-crash is extremely low, no one would suggest that taking two trips is a dangerous risk. These examples show the foolishness of taking small relative risks seriously.

Concerns about the state of epidemiology and the risks to public health from the abuse of language were raised almost three decades ago by Petr Skrabanek and his colleague James McCormick. They questioned whether epidemiology, in the absence of epidemics, was a misnomer for scaremongering, cloaked in sophisticated statistics.[6-8] They warned scientists to resist '*risk factorology*' – the practice of performing studies which relate a myriad of potential exposures to disease risk, and identifying those which are positively associated with disease as *risk-factors*, and those which are negatively linked as *protective-factors*. The practice continues today. In the absence of plausibility or hypothesis, researchers look for almost anything in the environment and our modern lifestyle that might affect human health. The number of variables is so high that the odds of finding a positive association are remarkably good. When results are positive, they are 'intriguing' and call for more research, and when negative, they are 'controversial' and call for more research. Either way, they get published. Danger to public health arises when risks are quoted only in relative, not absolute, terms and when any such association becomes transmuted to causation. For example, there is a high death rate associated with the intensive-care unit in most hospitals. This does not mean that intensive-care units kill people. One should not leap from correlation to causation.

MISLEADING MISNOMER

'Hygiene' is one of the most abused words in public health. Historically, clean water and proper sanitation have yielded remarkable improvements in public health. 'Cleanliness is next to godliness.' Perhaps! But hygiene is not the same as sterility. Humans co-evolved with tiny living creatures, known as microbes, and there are more microbes in and on the human body than human cells. So we are, in essence, only a minority component of ourselves! Human health is dependent on these microbes, because they educate the developing immune system and aid in the maturation of many human organs. However, in the 1980s, some scientists raised the possibility that excessive hygiene in modern societies with reduced childhood infections might be responsible for increasing rates of allergy and other chronic diseases. This became known as the 'hygiene hypothesis', and has been attributed to David Strachan, an English professor of epidemiology and population health, although the idea had already been fomented by others.

The hygiene hypothesis was conceptually appealing, seemed to fit with available data, but was wrong. The problem is not an obsession with public and personal hygiene. Rather, depletion of ancestral microbes due to overuse of antibiotics, and modern diets, probably accounts for the increasing frequency of allergies and other chronic diseases. The distinction is not a matter of semantics. Personal hygiene should not be abandoned. For example, hand-washing reduces the incidence of flu and other infections, some of which aggravate rather than reduce allergies and other chronic disorders. Mixed public health messages are confusing and difficult to erase, as shown by popular books with titles such as *Let Them Eat Dirt* or *Dirt is Good*.[3] For all their clever pithiness, these titles betray imprecise understanding of the now-abandoned hygiene hypothesis, and undermine public health efforts to constrain the spread of infectious diseases.[4] Moreover, these book titles have become seriously misplaced in a time of renewed focus on hand hygiene since the outbreak of Covid-19.

OBESITY: A PROBLEM DISTORTED BY BAD LANGUAGE AND LOGIC

In the summer of 2018, an unusual obituary of a sixty-four-year-old woman who died with cancer appeared in a Canadian newspaper.[5] The accompanying photograph, taken one week before her death, was chosen by her because she 'looked so good for someone almost dead!' Diagnosed with inoperable cancer days before her death, she had sought medical attention years earlier, but 'no one offered any support or suggestions beyond weight loss'. Whether the delayed diagnosis of cancer was related to doctors' attitudes to patients who are overweight will never be known, but her intent was to make people aware of the suffering that 'fat-shaming' can cause. Her dying wish was that 'women of size' make her death matter by advocating strongly for their health, and not accept fat as the only relevant health issue.

Considerable evidence points toward bias against overweight people throughout society, including health services. In many instances, doctors may be unaware of their bias, but prejudice is evident in the language they use. In Britain, a Health Minister actually urged health-care providers to tell patients who are obese that they are 'fat' rather than 'obese' to motivate them to take responsibility for their lifestyles.[6] The logic behind this ministerial pronouncement was not only flawed, it was counterproductive and stigmatising. A survey of over a thousand Americans looked at language used to express negative attitudes towards patients who are overweight. Participants were asked to rate ten commonly used terms for weight as desirable, stigmatising, blaming, or motivating to lose weight, and how they would react if stigmatised by their doctor's reference to their weight. The terms 'weight' and 'unhealthy weight' were rated most desirable, and the terms 'unhealthy weight' and 'overweight' were the most motivating to lose weight. However, terms like 'morbidly obese', 'fat' and 'obese' were rated most undesirable, stigmatising and blaming. Moreover, about 20 percent of participants reported that they would not attend future medical appointments if they felt stigmatised by a doctor's language.[7]

Most people with a chronic disorder would dislike being defined in language by that disorder. Person-first language is generally advocated ('the person with leprosy' not 'the leper'), and has been adopted widely, but seemingly not when it comes to obesity. For example, a literature search on Google Scholar reveals twenty times more references to 'people with diabetes' than 'diabetic people'. The opposite applies to obesity: the same kind of search yields fifteen times more references to 'obese people' than 'people with obesity'.

Obesity has become the world's biggest public health threat. Complications of obesity include diabetes, cardiovascular disease liver disease, high blood pressure, liver disease, increased risk of cancer, osteoarthritis, and poor self-esteem. These are beginning to overrun health services, divert resources from other pressing needs, and place a huge financial burden on society. With such a huge threat, one might anticipate a concerted, well-planned, multi-faceted strategy for management and prevention. Not so. Instead, there has been a stream of mixed signals, misleading messages, incoherent policies and silo-ed thinking. At a simplistic level, overweight and obesity has been framed as a discrepancy between energy (calorie) intake and expenditure (by exercise). In other words, it's the patient's fault: overconsumption and sloth. Eat less and move more is the simple solution. This leaves the individual stigmatised and guilt-laden. However, the energy-in/energy-out formula for weight regulation is only a half-truth, and a huge over-simplification that fails to take into account individual susceptibilities, food policies and obesogenic environments and lifestyles, such as the widespread use of energy-dense processed foods, reduction in home cooking, the growth in consumption of fast foods, the increasing popularity of eating out in restaurants, and reduced physical activity. In many cases, the obesogenic exposure begins in childhood and is beyond the control of an innocent child.

Public health messages have lost effectiveness – if they ever had any. In some quarters, the public is beginning to view overweight as normal. The emphasis on sugar taxes and high-energy sugar-sweetened beverages (SSBs) misses a bigger point: that we need to reduce general caloric intake, regardless of sources. Moreover, the false hope fostered by diets which omit one class of food (for example, fats or carbs) is undermined by the failure to concede that the one feature common to all effective diet plans is overall calorie reduction, regardless of how it is achieved. Radical weight-loss plans are not as effective as gradual, modest long-term plans, and exercise alone will not lead to weight loss. Long-term dietary adjustments and physical fitness from exercise confer separate health benefits unrelated to weight loss. Continual confusion from mixed and inaccurate messages has compounded the problem of obesity.

Flawed Language and Failure to Combat Antibiotic Resistance

Antibiotics have changed our world. They are essential to modern medicine. In addition to treating previously fatal infections like tuberculosis and pneumonia, antibiotics have made it possible for patients to undergo surgery successfully; they have made childbirth safer for mother and baby, and protect patients with weakened immunity, including those on chemotherapy for cancer. We have had the use of antibiotics for the past sixty years, but if predictions are correct, we will soon face a world without antibiotics. An increasing number of bacteria and other infectious microbes have become resistant to anti-microbial drugs, and the pipeline for inventing new drugs is drying up.

The campaign for antibiotic conservation is a bit like the struggle against global warming. As the polar ice melts away, politicians, who have never been known for long-range thinking, debate deadlines for others to meet. Similarly, public health officials and policymakers plead for reform of antibiotic prescribing practices, but clinicians deal with problems of the present in individual patients, not populations. It is time to direct the educational narrative on antibiotics towards the consumer, and time to make the message personal, not abstract. Messages focused on the overuse of antibiotics with resistance, leading to fewer treatment options for infections, are abstract, and have limited impact, since each individual is being asked to consider the greater good. The threat of global warming has shown how campaigns appealing to the better nature of individuals do not guarantee changes in societal behaviour.

Instead of preaching the theoretical importance of conserving antibiotics for the welfare of future generations, the immediate and personal dangers of antibiotic consumption should be the message. Most people are aware of antibiotic-associated diarrhoea, and some may have heard of *Clostridium-difficile*-associated colitis following antibiotics, but few may know that antibiotic-induced disturbances of the normal indigenous microbes resident in and on the body (collectively known as the *microbiome*) represent a risk-factor for later development of chronic diseases, including allergies and obesity-related metabolic disorders. If doctors were to inform patients of such dangers, enthusiasm for antibiotic consumption, particularly for soft indications with little evidence for a benefit, might be tempered.

Although antimicrobial resistance is a public health emergency, control measures have been feeble, in part because the language used to describe the problem is unclear and lacks urgency. The lack of clarity in the language used has been confirmed by surveys in the United States and in the United Kingdom which reveal remarkable misconceptions among the public, many of whom think it is the person, rather than the infecting organism, which becomes resistant.[8] The lack of urgency of public health messages regarding antimicrobial resistance is evident in the failure to make the infectious nature of the problem explicit. Health officials have been slow to appreciate that antimicrobial resistance may be a highly contagious infectious disease, and ultimately a threat to everyone. Some bacteria readily spread their resistance to antibiotics to other bacteria, and from one person to another. In many countries, patients are now screened for the presence of bacteria in their faeces that are resistant to the antibiotic carbapenem (carbapenem-resistant enterobacteriaceae, or CPEs). To be CPE-positive is a new stigma in healthcare, given to us by the healthcare system.

CHANGING THE NARRATIVE ON VACCINATION

People who deny the benefits of vaccines threaten the health of the entire population. However, trying to convince vaccine-deniers of the safety and effectiveness of vaccination is like trying to debate with conspiracy theorists, flat-earth enthusiasts and those who insist that Elvis is still alive. Vaccine-deniers will frequently resort to a belief held with religious-like fervour that doctors, scientists, government and the pharmaceutical companies are linked in a web of deception. Scientific data are dismissed as collusion among the vested interests. Instead, the vaccine-sceptics offer irrational arguments bolstered by anecdotes, half-truths, fragmentary evidence or truths taken out of context. Sadly, inaccurate statements by vaccine-deniers receive wide publicity when they are endorsed by fake experts and ill-informed celebrities. As pointed out by the award-winning science journalist Michael Specter, these people are a serious threat to public health, and cannot be ignored or dismissed as a marginal group of cranks. An internet search for the word *vaccination* in America will quickly yield not only the Centers for Disease Control but also the National Vaccine Information Center, which sounds like a government-sponsored agency but is actually the opposite. It is the website for 'the most powerful anti-vaccine organisation in America', according to Specter.

Logic and rational discussion does not appear to work with vaccine-deniers. Repeated assurance of safety seldom shifts their opinion, and may even be counter-productive. Unfortunately, the vaccine-deniers cannot be ignored, because infectious diseases are not solely individual health concerns; they are a matter of public health. Unvaccinated citizens within society represent a threat to the entire population. Attempts to eradicate infectious diseases such as measles were once a realistic aspiration for the World Health Organisation but have been derailed because rates of vaccination have been insufficient.

Cases of measles have increased in the United States in recent years because of parents refusing to vaccinate their children. In a 2015 study aimed at countering anti-vaccination attitudes published in the *Proceedings of the National Academy of Sciences USA*,[9] investigators showed that informing parents of the dangers of measles itself was more effective in changing anti-vaccination opinions than debating the merits or safety of the vaccine. In relation to parents' fear that the measles vaccine might cause autism in their children, direct reassurances failed to shift their attitudes. Parents need to hear the facts about measles, which have been documented over the centuries, long before vaccines were developed, and then they will know that by choosing not to vaccinate their loved ones, they are actually putting them at risk rather protecting them from autism. By choosing not to vaccinate their children, they are also putting other children at risk – the children of their friends and neighbours – because failure to vaccinate diminishes *herd immunity*.

Herd immunity refers to the immunity (vaccination status) of those around you: the herd. An unvaccinated individual within a herd that is immune because of vaccination is protected, because nobody can spread the infection. The herd protects the individual. But if vaccination rates within the herd drop below 90 percent, herd immunity diminishes and infections can spread. Some vulnerable children who are born with an immune deficiency disease, or those who are too young to be vaccinated, actually depend on herd immunity for protection. The concept was succinctly summarised by the essayist Eula Biss: 'Vaccination works by enlisting a majority in the protection of a minority.' Mass vaccination is far more effective than individual vaccination because of herd immunity. So, the public health narrative needs to convey the message that for public health to work for the individual, it must be a collective enterprise, and irrational fears of vaccines need to be supplanted by real messages of what happens when real diseases are allowed to spread.

Weary from Awareness

Everyday life is awash with information promoting awareness of diseases and dangerous behaviours. Making people aware of what it is like to have a disease or disability has value in breaking down stigma and discrimination. It may also help recruit public support for research and services. However, the news media have become crowded with awareness campaigns competing for attention. In many cases, the messages are diluted and ineffective, reach the wrong audience or, in some cases, are actually counterproductive. This leads to wastage and diversion of resources from higher priorities. In some cases, what appears to be a promotion of awareness is really advertising by another name. For example, one pharmaceutical company peddling a remedy for a common ailment announced that a survey funded by the same company had revealed that a high percentage of the population is 'suffering in silence', and encouraged the sufferers to consult their doctor to ask about a solution. Juxtaposed with this news item was an advertisement for a product for the same ailment.

Moreover, it is easy for politicians and celebrities to endorse mindless awareness campaigns, but simply providing information to raise awareness does little to change behaviour. There are many reasons why people do what they do, but lack of awareness or knowledge of the danger of their actions is well down the list. Smoking, alcohol and driving at speed show this. A huge gulf exists between awareness of a potential problem and motivation to do something about it, or to change behaviour to avoid it. Raising awareness about how common a bad health behaviour is, may actually make it worse by unwittingly providing an excuse: 'Well, everyone is doing it.' We need to be wary of awareness campaigns that lack strategies based on knowledge of social norms and behavioural intervention methods. A continual avalanche of awareness messages without effective behavioural change is merely an illusion of public health education.

12

⚜⚜⚜

The Patient and the System

'Impenetrability! That's what I say.'
—Humpty Dumpty to Alice, *Through the Looking Glass*
Politico-speak – Forbidden Words – Preferred Words – Words of Deflection
– Gobbledegook – Patient v. System – The Sophisticated Deception

An object within a 'system so total and overwhelming that we often mistake it for the world' is how essayist and poet Anne Boyer described herself when she was diagnosed with breast cancer. Her concept of the system as a series of interlocking systems is not unlike the self-perception of many clinicians as cogs within an enormous machine. No longer are doctors cast as agents of their patients; more than ever they serve as agents of the State in publicly funded systems, or as agents of the Medical Industrial Complex in privately funded systems.[1]

For all their variability and continual change, the one constant at the heart of all systems of healthcare is the patient-doctor relationship. Preservation of the patient-doctor relationship is considered critical for the future of healthcare, but support for that relationship by the system's bureaucracy is dubious.[2] Patients need more time, not more technology from their doctors. Doctors also need more time with patients for many reasons, not least of which is job satisfaction and avoidance of the modern affliction: burnout. Increasingly, patients with complex chronic or multiple diseases will need doctors to fulfil a role more akin to that of a head coach, assisted by specialist nurses and other healthcare professionals, advocating healthful behaviour and co-ordinating safe passage through the system. However, the system is surrounded by opaque and occasionally deceptive language.

POLITICO-SPEAK

Anyone who doubts the importance of language in manipulating public opinion regarding healthcare should look at how the Republicans opposed President Obama's universal healthcare plan in the USA. Working on behalf of the Republicans was Frank Luntz, a professional pollster and wordsmith: 'It's not what you say, it's what people hear', according to Luntz. Luntz uses focus-groups to test which words resonate with voters and to evaluate words and phrases which appear synonymous but which, in fact, are perceived differently by the public. Opponents would claim that Luntz's role was to select words that make the Republicans sound like they care about healthcare reform when they don't. Luntz produced a strategy document listing words and language to discredit the healthcare policy of the Democrats and to camouflage the inadequacies and incoherence of Republican policy.

Luntz also coached the Republicans to frame the nation's healthcare in terms of a threat posed by the Democrats: 'a Washington takeover'. The arguments against the Democrats were to focus on 'politicians and bureaucrats' rather than on the 'free market, tax incentives or competition'. The essence of the plan was not to frame the debate in terms that the Democrats were using but to use words that conveyed the opposite messages. He encouraged Republicans to 'humanise' their approach and to 'individualise' and 'personalise' rather than generalise, and to present the Democrats' plan in terms of time delays ('Delayed care is denied care'). High cost of healthcare was to be addressed in terms of tackling 'waste, fraud and abuse', whereas healthcare quality was to be equated to 'getting the treatment you need when you need it', rather than support delays involved in the Democrats' plan.

FORBIDDEN WORDS

Politicians like to control the language used by their employees and by the press. Although they will rarely, if ever, use the word 'censorship', they find it difficult to resist censoring official documents. One tends to think of censorship in corrupt countries, dictatorships, and tyrannical or backward societies, and in bygone centuries. However, censorship continues even in the most socioeconomically developed countries on earth. On 15 December 2017, the *Washington Post* reported that President Donald Trump and his administration had banned the following words from government documents related to the budget for the Centers for Disease Control and Prevention (CDC): *vulnerable, entitlement, diversity, transgender, fetus, evidence-based* and *science-based*. Alternative phrases were offered for some of these words. This was picked up by many news media and medical journals, and the National Academy of Sciences in the USA quickly issued a statement

THE PATIENT AND THE SYSTEM 167

expressing deep concern, particularly at the reported ban on 'evidence-based' and 'science-based' terms. While the ban related to budgetary documents, the message from the White House, and the attempted political interference in medical science, seemed clear. Although the acting director of the CDC was forced to respond to the uproar, and claimed that 'there were no banned words at CDC', the reported diktat was strangely Orwellian.

PREFERRED WORDS

Manipulating public opinion with words of deception, evasion, distraction, obfuscation and occasional lies, is not new. Politicians and bureaucrats have been doing it for as long as we have had politicians and bureaucrats. While professing policies of openness, transparency and accountability, most modern healthcare systems are supported by press secretaries, media consultants, public relations officers and spin-doctors, who often see their role as protecting the system from the public rather than accurately informing the public.

There is a language preferred by politicians: a series of jingles and bridging strategies to be used when they can't think of what to say but want to give a positive impression. Abstract concepts like 'health care expenditure' and 'resource allocation models' and 'personnel deployment' are favoured because they give the impression of authority and control when, in fact, they are usually bluster without substance. Promised new and improved health services don't actually begin; they *take time* and are *rolled out,* giving the impression of progression, with any delays understandably part of a phased plan.

Comfort-words for health ministers are easily recognised because they are seldom used by ordinary people, and tend to be deliberately vague and imprecise. These are the weasel words that allow for plausible deniability later, when the politician is cornered. They cater for the claim that the words have been misconstrued or taken out of context. Examples include the R-words: *review, reconfigure, reorganise* and *reform.* Politicians can safely promise *reform* of the service – which sounds innocuous and vaguely like progress, but may do more harm than good.

On the folly of reform and reorganisation without good reason, it has all been said before. The sentiment is eloquently summarised in the following quotation, often attributed to the Roman satirist Gaius Petronius, but probably from Charlton Ogburn Jr (1911-98), in *Harper's Magazine,* 'Merrill's Marauders: The truth about an incredible adventure' (Jan 1957):

> We trained hard, but it seemed that every time we were
> beginning to form up into teams, we would be reorganised.
> I was to learn later in life that we tend to meet any new
> situation by reorganising; and a wonderful method it can be
> for creating the illusion of progress while producing confusion,
> inefficiency, and demoralisation.

Continual restructuring of any organisation is expensive, time-
consuming and demoralising for staff. In healthcare, it may cost lives.
The Francis report on the Mid-Staffordshire tragedy, in which patients
died as a result of poor care and the failings of staff at two British hospitals
between 2005 and 2009, commented that continual reorganisation was
a contributory factor because it meant that managers were uncertain of
their roles and this led to poor performances.[3]

Why do organisations undergo the disorganisation of repeated
reorganisation? This question was addressed by an irreverent,
but nonetheless serious, systematic review of reasons for repeated
reorganisations; the most common was 'no good reason'.[4] Simply stated,
'where it is not necessary to change, it is necessary not to change'.[5]
Patients and their carers should be protected from ill-considered
change-experiments dressed up as reform.

Other words and concepts that appeal to politicians include the
process of *consultation with the key stakeholders.* This is usually either
a delaying tactic, or code for something that is done *after* a decision
has already been made internally, and consultation is undertaken
on sufferance, to give the appearance of wider inclusiveness. When it
comes to the matter of the cost of services, politicians don't speak of
spending, because that reminds us that it is taxpayers' money that is
being spent, and draws the next question, on value for money. Instead,
the preferred political-speak is *investment.* Likewise, they dislike using
hard numbers, such as the number of hospital beds required to deal
with waiting lists. The preferred term is *bed-capacity issues,* which is
suitably vague, and could refer to the efficiency of turnover of the same
number of beds.

Verbs seem to be danger-words for politicians. In contrast to
the world of marketing, where verbs are the action-words in the art
of persuasion (*'Just do it'* or *'I'm lovin' it'*), such words are cautiously
avoided in political-speak. As pointed out by broadcaster John
Humphrys, verbs commit the speaker. Soundbites like 'Delivering a
safer, more effective health service' (who is?) or 'Better health, better

future' (how?), or 'A policy for safer healthcare for all', are vaguely promising but mean very little, because they don't commit the speaker in a specific manner. Without a verb, there is no commitment. When a verb is used by a politician, it tends to be passive, and buried in an anodyne statement that places the speaker one step removed from a key commitment. For example, the health minister is unlikely to say: 'I will increase the number of hospital beds in the system.' Instead, he or she is more likely to say: 'I will commission a review of our bed-capacity issues to address gaps in the system.'

Some words for politicians are to be avoided at all costs. Words like *poverty*, which has a dominant influence on health, are particularly difficult for politicians, because they strike at core policies and failures of government, for which the politicians have no answer. Another word that politicians and health service executives dislike is *inequality,* which draws attention to the fact that the distribution of spending on health is not equal across different geographic sectors or socioeconomic groups. *Crisis* within the health service is never acknowledged; those who do use the word are accused of being *alarmist* and *shroud-waving;* politicians will reassure us that the situation is being *monitored.* Problems within the health services are never *problems*, they are *challenges*. Essentials for improvement are not accepted forthwith, they are things that can be *looked at* in the future.

Words of Deflection

In anticipation of being cornered on distasteful topics, like delayed services and hospital waiting times, politicians and managers usually have a collection of stock phrases. Reframing the question allows the problem to be deflected elsewhere: 'This is not really about hospital waiting lists; it's about moving care to the community.' Alternatively, the question may be deflected to someone else ('I have set up a task force to address this') or to the future ('I have commissioned a report'). Even matters of urgency may be deflected ('Let's not make rash decisions; it would be imprudent to pre-empt the forthcoming report'). When pressed on timelines, specific dates are deflected to a hope that it will be done 'as soon as possible', with the secret preference that it can be spun out for as long as possible, or at least until it becomes someone else's problem. Finally, there is deflection to the past, by acknowledging all that has been done already, while graciously thanking those who have worked hard on the issue and conceding that 'more needs to be done' – without specifying by whom. There are also the ploys of blaming current deficiencies on what has been inherited from the previous government, and avoiding probing questions with bland statements like 'This government is investing more in our health service than ever before'.

GOBBLEDEGOOK

We know it when we hear it. No explanation required. It is immediately recognisable, adopted enthusiastically by politicians and their officials: verbose bluster intended to give the illusion of deliberative action. Its popularity is reflected by the number of names for it: *raiméis* in Ireland; *mumbo-jumbo, blather, gibberish* and *poppycock* in the UK. It is known everywhere as *gobbledegook*. The word was first used by Maury Maverick, a politician from Texas, to describe attempts by speakers or authors to impress their listeners or readers, but actually presenting an image of a strutting turkey (*gobble-gobble, gobble-gobble*).

The absurdity of governmental gobbledegook was mercilessly lampooned in the BBC television sitcom of the 1980s, *Yes Minister*, written by Jonathan Lynn and Antony Jay. The great success of the show was that it created humour that was rooted in fact, and changed the way the public looked at the political world. Many of the episodes not only reprised actual events in real life, but also anticipated future ones. Perhaps the most memorable episode concerned the story of the hospital with no patients. The Civil Service officials defended the hospital, claiming that 'It takes *time* to get things going . . . to sort out the smooth running of the hospital. Having *patients* around would be no help at all. . . . They'd just be in the way.' The Minister becomes exasperated when the administrators seem unperturbed by the costs of maintaining a facility while it is not being used:

> '*But there are no patients!*' exclaims the Minister.
> 'No-o-o, but the essential work of the hospital still has to go on.'
> '*Aren't patients the essential work of the hospital?*'
> 'Oh, running an organisation of five hundred people is a *big* job, Minister.'

The episode has been used to remind bureaucrats that they should be more concerned about outcomes rather defending their Department at all costs. It also highlighted how dependent politicians are on their officials, and how resistant these officials are to change. The best lines in the sitcom were given to the canny permanent secretary of the Department, Sir Humphrey, who was a long-term survivor of many different political administrations. For example, the Minister complains that the hospital without patients is symbolic of the malaise affecting public policy: 'The National Health Service, Humphrey, is an advanced case of galloping bureaucracy!' The experienced Sir Humphrey calmly responds: 'Oh, certainly not galloping. A gentle *canter* at the most!'

Sir Humphrey represents civil-service-speak. He is a master of loquacious words of wisdom; he knows how to obfuscate, and how to maintain plausible deniability. Most importantly – and as with all bureaucracies – he clings to the status quo and is primarily concerned with self-preservation. He dislikes decisions. In his world, decisions are not necessarily decisions; a decision may merely be 'the course the Minister seems to favour at the moment'.

One of the words that health-service bureaucrats continually abuse is *leadership*. The distinction between a leader and a manager becomes lost, and the two words are often used interchangeably. Managers dislike being reminded that leaders set policy, whereas managers effect policy, not the other way round. In recent years, a new term, the clinical *lead*, has crept into medical administrative parlance. The clinical *lead* is a clinician who has influence and responsibility for a particular area of the medical service, but usually without power to do much about it. It seems that two thirds of the word (*lead-* without the *-er*) is somehow less threatening. A medley of fashionable bureau-speak jingles in current parlance is listed in the table below.

Health-system-speak	Plain-speak interpretation
Bed capacity	Number of beds
Resource implications	Will cost us
Resources	Money, people or time, or all three
Investment	Spend money (no one invests in their garden or their house or their car: they buy things with money)
International best practice	Something copied from elsewhere
Strategic planning group	A committee
Task force	Another committee
Working group	Yet another committee
Stakeholders	People who care
Vested interests	Blame the doctors and nurses
A safe pair of hands in control	A dead hand

Health-system-speak	Plain-speak interpretation
Centre of excellence	Just a centre
A premature leak to the media	A strategy to sample public opinion in advance of unveiling a dodgy policy or decision
Consultation with stakeholders	To give the appearance of inclusiveness after a decision has been made by others; to suffer the comments and then ignore them

Of course, gobbledegook is not always intended as a deception. It is generally a benign form of bad language, related to lazy thinking and inflated by jargon, abbreviations and clichés. Technobabble pervades many organisations, and is never acceptable, but it becomes dangerous when clarity of communication is critical, as in a health service. It is particularly disappointing when it comes from those who should know better, at the top of the organisation. Consider the introductory paragraph of a communiqué which was widely circulated by the director general of one of the health services in which I have worked:

> Dear Colleagues,
> You will be aware that as an integral part of our journey to build a better health service, the National Centre Transformation Programme, which commenced in 2015 under my sponsorship, continues to be one of the main drivers for the transformation of the National Centre.

This would appear to reassure the reader that his transformation programme in the centre is the main driver of transformation in the centre, but just to be sure:

> Notwithstanding these recent changes, it is my intention to continue in the role of overall sponsor of the National Centre Transformation Programme, reflecting the importance of this work. I have commenced a process to review the component elements of the programme to ensure that it maintains a focus on delivering on its object to transform the corporate centre with a primary focus on enabling and empowering a strong delivery system which is apparently resourced, empowered and accountable for making decisions and delivering services closer to the population.

No doubt there were noble intentions here, some even quite sensible, but lost in lazy language. The memo ran for three pages, and included a plan of distinct phases of activity, including an additional 'plan for the transition approach' to 'assess the impact and commence the process of implementing the changes', thereby undermining the first sentence, which claimed that the changes were already under way. Six days later, the same director general launched a document entitled: 'Guidelines for Communicating Clearly Using Plain English with Our Patients and Service Users'.[6]

Patient v. System

Charles Dickens' description of the circumlocution office, written over a hundred and fifty years ago, is still a familiar image of what many are faced with when they seek help by engaging with government bureaucracy, including a national health service:

> The Circumlocution Office . . . the most important Department under government . . . half a score of boards, half a bushel of minutes, several sacks of official memoranda, and a family-vault-full of ungrammatical correspondence, on the part of the Circumlocution Office. . . . It being one of the principles of the Circumlocution Office never. . . [to] give a straightforward answer.
>
> —Charles Dickens, *Little Dorrit,* 1857[7]

One has to be in a position of privilege to penetrate much of the language of bureaucracy, and even then, persistence is required. Moreover, according to Theodore Dalrymple (aka Dr Anthony Daniels), 'it is patently untrue that every man's language is equal to his needs, a fact that is obvious to anyone who has read the pitiable attempts of the underclass to communicate in writing with others, especially officialdom'. Equality is an aspiration of most health services, including the British National Health Service, but amongst the hidden inequities is the differential response of officialdom to the linguistic skills of patients. According to Dalrymple, the educated middle classes 'know better how to take advantage of what the system offers': they are more articulate, vociferous and argumentative.

The work of Ken Loach, British filmmaker and champion of the disadvantaged, has explored the complexity of literacy, and how it influences what the vulnerable and the poor must endure when they attempt to engage with officialdom. Loach's award-wining movie *I, Daniel Blake* (2016) tells the story of a fifty-nine-year-old woodworker and widower who has been forced out of work following a heart attack and, while he is recovering, finds himself at war with two disconnected governmental bureaucracies, one medical and the other employment-based. Reminiscent of Dickens' circumlocution office, Loach's fictional story is full of the evasive language, euphemisms and multiplying absurdities of a system where digital dialogue has replaced human contact. What human contact Daniel manages to make is equally evasive and non-committal.

Daniel's nightmare begins when, acting on his doctor's orders not to return to manual work, he applies for disability allowance. The application is rejected because of his responses to a series of inane questions ('Can you raise either arm to the top of your head . . . put a hat on your head . . . press a button?'). He is deemed fit for work by the system's official assessor, described as a 'healthcare professional', and his complaint ('You've got me medical records . . . I wanna get back to work . . . Can we just talk about me heart?') is ignored. This is followed by a series of frustrated appeals and unsuccessful attempts on the phone to make contact with a human being within the system. The absurdities of the system multiply when he is forced to apply for jobseeker's allowance, which requires that he seek work – which, if offered, he must decline. In one heart-rending scene, Daniel, who has never used a computer, is forced into a pathetic attempt to complete an application form online.

The coldness of the system, with its inadequate heartless language ('digital by default') is contrasted with the simplicity of Daniel's words ('pencil by default'). He is disadvantaged by his lack of computer literacy, but his innate decency and kindness towards another, who is worse off, shows the value of people caring for people, and what the system had denied him.

Stories of patients' experiences with the healthcare system can reveal more than statistics. Dr Faith Fitzgerald described the contrasting experiences of two patients with the same complaint (diarrhoea) who were managed within the same year but by two different healthcare systems. The first was her elderly mother, who endured delays, insensitivity bordering on rudeness, and a hefty bill for inconclusive postponed investigations. The second patient was a ten-year old male, also with diarrhoea, who was seen promptly, greeted warmly, investigated immediately, and inexpensively, and treated with respect and kindness. Were the differences attributable to age discrimination or just a bad day for the first system? No: the second patient, her dog, was treated by a veterinarian healthcare system.

THE SOPHISTICATED DECEPTION

Jaded by false promises and decades of unfulfilled policies, modern society is alert to the language of deception, but some of the language-manipulation in healthcare is particularly cunning, and not obvious to the unsuspecting public. Consider the publicity surrounding patient-satisfaction surveys. Frequently, the official response to failures in public healthcare is to defend the indefensible by invoking results of a patient-satisfaction survey claiming that most patients are happy with the care they receive in hospital. How often do we hear officialdom claim that 'the system works well because surveys show that most people are happy with the care they have received'! The deception here is that customer-service surveys, particularly patient-satisfaction surveys, routinely return high levels of satisfaction.[8]

Firstly, patient satisfaction surveys are usually conducted after an acute admission to hospital or after some form of treatment, and ignore those who are waiting for treatment or have not been able to access it. Secondly, the results of surveys are often in striking contrast with the accounts that patients give to friends and family. In fact, many patients despair at the prospect of complaining, and feel they are being fobbed off. Even patients who have responded positively in a satisfaction questionnaire convey a different story on subsequent direct questioning. They dislike blaming front-line medical and nursing staff for bad experiences, feeling it was 'not their fault', or express sympathy for the conditions under which staff are expected to work. Negative experiences are quickly forgotten or forgiven if the overall outcome is good. Many patients who respond positively in a satisfaction survey actually feel that their treatment was similar to that of others, and 'it's the best you can expect from the system'.

In a historical review of the doctor-patient relationship (*Bedside Manners*), Professor Edward Shorter at the University of Toronto wrote that 'Patients are willing to declare themselves happy with the most appalling medical service; so much do they hope they've been given good care that they are seldom able to face the prospect that they haven't.'

Reports of high satisfaction should not be assumed to reflect good experiences in relation to medical services. The benchmark should be levels of negative experience, and surveys should be renamed, and results expressed, in terms of dissatisfaction scores.

13

⋘⋘⋘

The Language of Plagues and Pandemics

'Virus: bad news wrapped in protein'

—Peter Medawar

Pandemic Parlance – Finding the Personal stories – Misnomers and Metaphors – Binary Language and Logic – A Communications Emergency – A Pandemic Pause To Consider Our Place in Nature

'Unprecedented' said the politicians and pundits, accounting for a lack of preparedness for Covid-19. Who could have predicted such a thing? But it wasn't unprecedented, and it was predicted. Plagues and pandemics have shaped human history through the ages. Experts say that when you've seen one pandemic, you've seen . . . one pandemic. Pandemics differ because microbes differ. Context and the vulnerability of populations also vary.

There are, of course, parallels and lessons to be learned from all pandemics. First, there is the naming and blaming. Then there is the stigmatisation and marginalisation of minorities, and eventually pandemics reveal societal and healthcare inequities. Pandemics are communications emergencies as well as health and economic threats. Leadership during pandemics is valued as much for clear and consistent messages as for decisiveness. Survivors look for meaning. They may wonder about our place in nature and ask: who is in control, microbes or mankind?

Pandemic Parlance

One of the first casualties of Covid-19 was non-verbal communication. Hugs, handshakes and human touch disappeared. Kindness was difficult to express from two metres, or from behind masks and goggles. Another casualty was the infection of pandemic parlance with fake news and false facts. The World Health Organisation has been fighting a pandemic *and* an *infodemic*, defined as a flood of misinformation, disinformation and opinion, spreading faster than the virus.

Pandemics also change the way people speak. The 'new normal' of Corona-speak included slogans and soundbites rallying everyone to 'come together by staying apart'. 'Flattening the curve', 'social distancing', and searching for 'super-spreaders' and 'second spikes' became part of the language, but 'personal protective equipment' (PPE) still sounds as clumsy as it is to wear. 'Lockdown' and 'cytokine storm' invoke memories of climatic crises. Then there is waiting for the 'endgame' (vaccination) and 'herd immunity', but 'zoonosis' (infection acquired from animals) is likely to be remembered only by people who play Scrabble.

Pandemic words are not new; they describe established public health concepts. However, ordinary words like *essential, necessary, elective, urgent* and *emergent* acquire added significance during a pandemic. No one disputed the need to cancel elective operations to conserve hospital resources during the Covid-19 crisis. But *elective* does not mean *unnecessary* or *non-essential.* An elective operation for curable cancer is essential, whereas cosmetic surgery is elective and non-essential. What should a doctor say to a patient when an essential operation is postponed because it is elective? When does *essential* turn into *urgent*? How long a wait must there be until a curable cancer becomes incurable because of postponement? The fickle nature of words is seldom appreciated by decisionmakers distant from the frontline, but it may jeopardise the welfare of non-Covid patients.

Numbers are as important as words in pandemics. Epidemiology is like economics; it deals with numbers, a language of diseases within populations, not illness in individuals. Contagious diseases are recorded as *outbreaks* (regional increase in affected cases), *epidemics* (large numbers of people affected within a population) and *pandemics* (global spread). When a problem persists in a specific location, it is said to be *endemic.*

The two most important numbers during a pandemic or any health scare are the *numerator* (e.g. the number of deaths) and the *denominator* (total number of affected cases). Too often the numerator is given without the denominator, but this alone is impossible to interpret properly, and is not comparable from one population to another. Calculating the death-rate requires knowledge of both numbers. Likewise, when politicians claim to be doing more testing than any other country, the total number of tests (numerator) is meaningless without knowing the total population (denominator).

'Test, test, test', a Covid-19 slogan from WHO, prompted politicians and administrators to announce total numbers of tests performed as if it were an international contest. However, the total number of tests is almost meaningless without context, such as the number of tests

178 THE LANGUAGE OF ILLNESS

per day, and the turnaround time from testing to receiving a result. In order to be effective, test results must come quickly, and be available to healthcare professionals as soon as possible.

The R-number (reproduction number) is the average number of people to whom one infected person passes the virus. In other words, it is a measure of the spread of the virus. Factors that influence the R-value include human behaviour, the length of time one remains infectious, the resistance (immunity) of the population, the population density, and the way by which the virus spreads (airborne illnesses spread faster than those which require direct contact). Measles and influenza have a high R-value, whereas that for hepatitis C is relatively low. Changing human behaviour by physical isolation can push the R-value to less than 1, in which case the disease declines; if the R-value drifts above 1, there may be secondary spikes.

FINDING THE PERSONAL STORIES

Behind the numbers are people and their stories. In Albert Camus' novel *The Plague*, Dr Rieux wearily listens to the radio at night and hears 'kindly, well-meaning speakers' who try to voice their fellowship, 'but at the same time proved the utter incapacity of every man truly to share in suffering that he cannot see'.

Inexplicably, the suffering from the influenza pandemic of 1918-19 was hidden among the numbers dying and the obscenities of a raging world war. 'When the dying stopped, the forgetting began', it was said, after the horrors of the 1918 influenza pandemic in the United States. 'Collective amnesia' is how the Irish president and poet Michael D. Higgins described the manner in which the 1918-19 pandemic quickly receded from national consciousness until recent times. As memorials were erected around the globe to ensure that those fallen in battle should never be forgotten, those who fell in far greater numbers to the influenza pandemic seemed to drift from public memory. Survivors remembered in silence.

Historians assembled the shocking facts and statistics of the 1918 pandemic, and scientists uncovered the biological components and molecular mechanisms of the disease. However, personal accounts of the suffering were elusive. Where was the humanity among the facts? One of the lessons from 1918-19 is the need to hear patients' voices in contemporary accounts so that the scale of human suffering is not forgotten. What was it really like? How did it feel?

'Death steals everything,' wrote the poet Jim Harrison, 'except our stories.' In the novel *Look Homeward, Angel,* Thomas Wolfe told the story of his brother Ben dying from influenza. 'We can believe in the nothingness of life, we can believe in the nothingness of death and of life after death,' wrote Wolfe, 'but who can believe in the nothingness of Ben.'

Katharine Anne Porter's experience of near-fatal influenza led to her autobiographical novel *Pale Horse, Pale Rider*. This is the story of Miranda, a young woman who becomes seriously ill with influenza, and is nursed by her fiancé, who later dies from the illness. 'It's as bad as anything can be,' he tells her, 'all the theatres and nearly all the shops and restaurants are closed, and the streets have been full of funerals all day and ambulances all night.' At first, Miranda's symptoms seem ordinary, headaches and 'pain all over', but she has a dark foreboding ('There's something terribly wrong. . . . I feel too rotten' and 'Something terrible is going to happen to me'), and then a feeling of life slipping away:

> Almost with no warning at all, she floated into the darkness. . . . She sank easily through deeps and deeps of darkness until she lay like a stone at the farthest bottom of life, knowing herself to be blind, deaf, speechless, no longer aware of the members of her own body.

When all seemed hopeless, she began to recover with a 'stubborn will to live': 'pain returned . . . she opened her eyes and saw pale light . . . knew that the smell of death was in her own body, and struggled to lift her hand.' She looked about her 'with the covertly hostile eyes of an alien who does not like the country in which he finds himself, does not understand the language nor wish to learn it, does not mean to live there and yet is helpless, unable to leave it at his will.'

The aftermath was a 'dazed silence', perhaps a muted form of post-viral depression.

Porter's novel (which was first published in 1939) was unusual for its time. Most writers ignored influenza, despite the global impact the disease had in the early twentieth century. No one has been as effective as Porter in finding words for the personal suffering inflicted by influenza. However, the experience of illness has been expressed in other art-forms. Edvard Munch, who survived the influenza pandemic, captured a sense of isolation, post-viral despair and continuing infirmity in his *Self Portrait after the Spanish Flu (1919)*.

It would take almost a century before the individual stories of the influenza pandemic would re-emerge. Most historical analyses and fictional accounts of this disease appeared within the past two decades. In the popular television series *Downton Abbey* (Season 2, episode 8), three members of the house develop influenza. The death of Lavinia is shown with family members gathered around the bedside; her fiancé holding her hand as she slipped away. Death-scenes like this would have been daily realities in 1918-19, but stand in contrast with death in the time of Covid-19, when too many died alone, without the comfort of human touch, and survivors were left without the rituals of grieving together.

It is unclear why the 1918-19 influenza pandemic left so little cultural trace. It is even more difficult to imagine a time when the post-Covid-19 'new normal' gives way to complacency and amnesia. Individuals will remember the stories and losses of loved ones, but collectively, society quickly forgets.

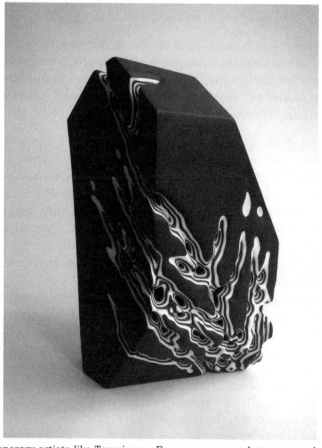

Contemporary artists like Tamsin van Essen use no words to convey the sense of a host being attacked by the creeping spread of a virus. Her porcelain pieces represent at once the beauty of the human form and its imperfections at the boundary between health and disease.
Image used with the kind permission of the artist.

MISNOMERS AND METAPHORS

Naming the enemy is standard war-time strategy, but as discussed throughout this book, mislabelling is hazardous. Repeated references to Covid-19 as the 'Chinese virus' unnecessarily increased international tension and put Asian-Americans at risk of racial slurs and abuse. Likewise, 'Spanish flu' was a misnomer for the 1918-19 pandemic. The origin of that pandemic is unknown. Spain's neutrality during World War I meant that its statistics for influenza were uncensored and it was unfairly linked with the outbreak.

Science now uses precise, non-racial terminology for viruses, but people and politicians prefer metaphors. 'Invisible enemy', 'great leveller', and a result of a 'perfect storm' quickly became metaphors for Covid-19. However, Covid-19 is an accidental enemy, not a malevolent one – the result of chance, time and human behaviour. Nor is it a leveller. Rather, it is a revealer of societal inequities, poor leadership and unpreparedness. Moreover, scientists argue that a 'perfect storm' is a simplistic and unsatisfactory explanation for the origin of Covid-19 because it invokes the notion of unpredictability and absence of human agency or social responsibility. Perfect-storm language conveniently ignores the contribution of human behaviour to the emergence and prevention of pandemics. The same is true of the 'Black Swan' metaphor when used in relation to the Covid pandemic. A Black Swan event is how Nassim Nicholas Taleb describes highly improbable economic events. The Black Swan is an 'outlier', without precedent to point to the possibility of its existence. Its impact is extreme, and humans contrive explanations for it *after* the fact in an attempt to make it predictable.

Not all pandemic metaphors are misplaced. The most popular is the war metaphor, which serves a useful purpose for rallying 'the troops', supporting doctors and nurses in 'the trenches' at the 'front line', under the dubious leadership of a 'war-time president' while the Queen invoked the spirit of World War II ('We will meet again'). In truth, pandemics are not wars. They represent a time when compassion, cooperation and aid are needed, not aggression and blame. Therefore, the language of an international emergency is preferable because it invokes humanitarianism, caring and kindness. The 'Covid emergency' is how the Irish Taoiseach (prime minister) referred to the crisis, recalling what was once the popular term for World War II ('the Emergency') in Ireland.

New York governor Andrew Cuomo used many metaphors to explain and simplify, and to rally New Yorkers to a common cause during the Covid-19 pandemic. In support of the use of facial masks, he cleverly turned the mask into a metaphor for societal solidarity: 'I wear a mask not to protect myself from getting the infection from you, but as a gesture to show that I want to protect you from getting the infection from me.'

BINARY LANGUAGE AND LOGIC

Over time, binary language becomes insufficient for describing human relationships with microbes. Simple designations like *contact* or *non-contact*, *infected* or *uninfected*, and *symptomatic* or *asymptomatic* carrier need greater nuance. As Dr Siddhartha Mukherjee points out, the measurement of a virus spreading *across* people should be supplemented with measurement of the virus *within* people. It is not enough to detect the presence or absence of the virus; rather, we need to know more about the viral load, or amount of virus in the body. With many infections, the dose of viral exposure and levels of the virus in the body determine the risk of infection and the severity of illness following infection. Just as the shape and peak of the curve of viral infections in the population is measured, it is also important to know the shape of the curve, and peak levels of virus, in an individual.

Similarly, binary language is not suited to the 'hard choices' leaders make in balancing science over economics, health or wealth, and lives or livelihoods. These are not real choices; they represent inseparable interdependent values, not alternatives. Pandemics are first and foremost health crises, which quickly become economic crises. However, there is no either/or, no 'cure that's worse than the disease' in managing a pandemic. Health and economics must be tackled together. Medical science has long recognised that there is more to health than healthcare, and that illness accompanies impoverishment.

Related to the problem of binary language is the flawed logic of the 'preparedness paradox'. This is a form of damned-if-you-do-and-damned-if-you-don't problem. It arose several times during the Covid-19 crisis, when proponents for 'opening up' the economy claimed that the public health advocates were overreacting. Sceptics claimed that the preventive measures must have been unnecessary, since the health services were not overrun. In other words, the success of the preparedness strategy was the basis of the criticism. 'People sometimes think that you're overreacting,' responded Dr Anthony Fauci, Director of the National Institute of Allergy and Infectious Diseases; 'I like it when people are thinking I'm overreacting, because that means we're doing it just right. '

A COMMUNICATIONS EMERGENCY

Cometh the hour, cometh the man . . . or woman. The inadequacies of political leaders are quickly found out by pandemics. Their responses to the Covid-19 crisis were not all bad and not all good. Most politicians were, at first, unprepared, but defining features of responsible leadership, much of it from women, included truthfulness, clear communication, consistent messages, and decisiveness. People look to their leaders in a time of crisis for information, support and direction. Clarity, transparency and consistency are essential for public trust. Without trust, there is fear and confusion. In Camus' *The Plague*, Dr Rieux asks if the journalist will be allowed to tell the truth. 'I mean,' Rieux explained, 'would you be allowed to publish unqualified condemnation of the present state of things?'

During the Covid-19 crisis, the US President displayed none of the required leadership characteristics. Presidential pronouncements were inaccurate, inconsistent and dangerous. International viewers were aghast at chaotic press conferences during which the President blamed others, insulted journalists and evaded questions. The absurdity prompted one American journalist to announce: 'The President just told us that he didn't tell us what he just told us.' Inconsistent messaging and hesitant intervention was also a feature of political leadership in the United Kingdom, which had to retreat from an initial policy of wishful thinking and watchful expectancy of herd immunity developing.

Slogans used by politicians during the Covid-19 pandemic were devised for simplicity and clarity. They also revealed much about healthcare systems. For example, in New York the Governor's banner was 'Stay home – Stop the spread – Save lives', whereas in the United Kingdom the corresponding slogan was 'Stay home – Protect the NHS – Save lives'. In contrast to the United States, which has a largely private hospital system, the UK has a publicly funded national healthcare system (the NHS). Sadly, the initial focus on protecting the system from being overrun, distracted attention from the most vulnerable in society. In particular, protection of nursing-home residents was unduly delayed. When it became clear that the NHS was not going to be overwhelmed, and when pressure mounted to re-open the economy, the British government changed its slogan to 'Stay alert – Control the virus – Save lives'. The change created a sense of ambiguity, inconsistency and a relaxation of control. 'Stay apart' would have been less vague than 'Stay alert', whereas 'Control the virus' confused many people and provided material for ridicule by comics.

Mistakes can be anticipated in crises. People are remarkably forgiving when mistakes are acknowledged, but will sense bluster and quickly resent concealment of truth. False promises regarding tests and protective equipment for Covid-19 eroded confidence in the pronouncements of the US administration. In the United Kingdom, a government spokesman, well coached in dealing with the media, resorted to defensive bureaucratic language when asked why front-line medical staff were left inadequately protected. Instead of simple language, evasive words were used. Instead of admitting there was a 'shortage' of masks, equipment and tests, he said there is a 'need for more'. Instead of admitting a 'problem' (with such shortages), he described it as a 'challenge'. Instead of apologising to the front-line workers, he said 'I'm sorry if people feel they can't get these items' – thereby deflecting responsibility for the situation.

A Pandemic Pause To Consider Our Place in Nature

Who is in control, mankind or microbe? Humans evolved with viruses, bacteria and other tiny creatures. We call them 'microbes' because we can't see them, but they are there all right, in and on the human body. Madonna sings about living in a material world, but it is a higher truth that we live in a *microbial* world:

> You know that we are living in a microbial world
> And I'm a microbial girl.

We share our world with microbes. Far from being at war with microbes, we depend on them. As discussed in Chapter 11, human health is dependent on a harmonious relationship with microbes. Moreover, mankind has used microbes to produce vital drugs, and everything from cleaning up oil slicks to botox.

Viruses are numerically the most successful biological entities on the planet. They pre-date human existence, and are a dominant driver of evolution and biodiversity in nature. Ancient viral DNA accounts for about 8 percent of the human genome. Humans contain vast numbers of viruses, greatly exceeding the numbers of human cells. Inescapably, a human is a superorganism: part *Homo sapiens* and part microbial.

As a cause of disease, most viruses are innocent, accidental culprits. Most of the viruses in humans control the numbers and composition of bacteria colonising the human body. Others, like the herpes simplex (cold sore) and zoster (shingles) viruses, take up residence in human cells and live in delicate balance with their host, emerging only when human immunity dips. It is seldom in a virus's interest to kill its host; deadly viruses like smallpox tend to be those which humans can eliminate or evade with a change in human behaviour.

When pandemic viruses come along, they remind us of the fragility and interconnectedness of life, and humankind's delicate relationship with nature. Like other microbes, pandemic viruses tell us much about human behaviour. To what degree did human behaviour contribute to the circumstances that allowed Covid-19 to emerge and spread? Reassuringly, the human response to pandemics is an opportunity to show what it means to be human. To date, the public response to Covid-19 seems to confirm what Camus' Dr Rieux concluded: 'in a time of pestilence . . . there are more things to admire in men than to despise.'

Epilogue

Someday, sooner or later, the reader will play a role in the illness-story of a loved one. The way you play that role can mitigate or accentuate the ordeal of illness. The experience of illness is unique, and cannot be generalised. This means that engaging with the ill needs time, and then more time.

What To Say . . . Or Not!

The language of illness – spoken or unspoken – is not complicated. Simple truths, silent presence and listening suffice. It begins with confronting our own awkwardness, and a determination not to indulge in self-serving contrivances that permit us to stay away.

How to behave with the ill
Don't ignore. Show that you care. Be there. Bear witness.
Get over your awkwardness with the ill. Confront and accept illness.
Don't be a minimiser, a philosopher, a storyteller or a peddler of remedies or received wisdom.
Kind words suffice, but words are not essential. No clichés.
'I don't know what to say' is the honest thing to say.
If invited, don't be afraid to touch. Everyone can use a hug.

Few doctors, nurses or other professional carers would concede a lack of awareness of the issues raised in this book. However, passive, distant awareness is insufficient; only active, engaged awareness counts. Testimony from doctors and nurses who get sick suggests that the experience of illness is an epiphany, revealing large gaps in awareness of the language of illness and how to behave with the ill. Maybe this explains why the science of medicine advances at pace, but the humanity of medicine does not.

Notes

CHAPTER 2: DOCTOR-SPEAK AND ITS DISTANCING EFFECT

1. Eliza Dolittle didn't say this in George Bernard Shaw's original play *Pygmalion* but she did sing it in the song 'Show Me' in the 1964 movie *My Fair Lady* (lyrics by Alan Jay Lerner and music by Frederick Loewe).

2. Bridge, Edward M. *The Language of Medicine: A Study of Medical Vocabulary.* The University of Buffalo, Buffalo, 1962. (Also published in abbreviated form in the *Journal of Medical Education,* March 1962;37:201-210.)

3. Smith, C. M. 'Origin and uses of *primum non nocere* – above all, do no harm!' *Journal of Clinical Pharmacology,* 2005;45:371-377.

4. Metrorrhagia is uterine bleeding at irregular intervals, particularly between menstrual periods. In other words, it is inter-menstrual bleeding. Menometrorrhagia is a combination of inter-menstrual bleeding (metrorrhagia) and heavy menstrual bleeding.

5. Crotchets: Kilpatrick, J. J. My crochets and your crotchets. In: *The Writers Art,* J. J. Kilpatrick. Andrews, McMeel & Parker, Kansas, New York, 1984; Hurst, J. W. 'Crotchets: bothersome attitudes, habits, opinions and language.' *Clinical Cardiology,* 1998; 21:544-46.; Hurst, J. W. 'Crotchets' (1999). *Clinical Cardiology,* 1999; 22, 611-613; McCartney, M. 'Bad language'. *British Medical Journal,* 2015; May 5;350:h2342. doi: 10.1136/bmj.h2342.; Richards, T., 2017, April 7. *BMJ Blogs* http://blogs.bmj.com/bmj/2017/04/07/tessa-richards-words-that-annoy-phrases-that-grate/

6. The Medical Record: Weed, L. L. *Medical Records, Medical Education and Patient Care.* The Press of Case Western Reserve University, Chicago, 1969; Weed, L. L, Weed, L., *Medicine in Denial.* Createspace, 2013. Scotts Valley, California.; Donnelly, W. J., 'Medical language as symptom: doctor talk in teaching hospitals'. *Perspectives on Biological Medicine.* 1986 Autumn; 30(1):81-94.; Donnelly, W. J. 'The language of medical case histories'. *Annals of Internal Medicine.* 1997;127:1045–8.; Donnelly, W. J. 'Enriching the case history'. *Academic Medicine.* 2000 Jul;75(7):677.; Donnelly, W. J. 'Viewpoint: patient-centered medical care requires a patient-centered

medical record.' *Academic Medicine*, 2005 Jan;80(1):33-38; Donnelly, W. J. 'Patients' stories as narrative'. *Journal of the American Medical Association*, 2002;287:447.

7.   Dr Seamus O'Mahony has criticised the hijacking of patients' stories under the rubric of 'narrative medicine', which has become imbued with unnecessary and obscure academic jargon. Moreover, he is critical of the sentimentality and consumerism linked with 'narratology', and disputes claims that narrative medicine can teach empathy. (O'Mahony, Seamus. 'Against narrative medicine'. *Perspectives in Biology and Medicine*, 2013;56:611-619.)

8.   *Medical Slang.* The author, Dr Stephen Bergman, has described why he wrote the book (Shem Samuel, *The House of God.* Black Swan, 1978, London) and has offered a perspective on the fortieth anniversary of its publication. Not much has changed. (Shem, S.: 'Fiction as resistance'. *Annals of Internal Medicine,* 2002;137;934-937; 'Basch Unbound: *The House of God* and Fiction as Resistance at 40'. *Journal of the American Medical Association,* 2019; published online only. Reviews of medical slang by other authors include the following: Fox, A. T., Fertleman, M., Cahill, P., Palmer, R. D. 'Medical slang in British hospitals'. *Ethics & Behavior,* 2003;13:173-189.; Keeley P. 'Pimp my slang'. *British Medical Journal,* 2007;335:1295, and Goldman B. *The Secret Language of Doctors: Cracking the Code of Hospital Culture.* Triumph Books, Chicago, 2014.

9.   Not the full shilling: In 1971, the UK and Ireland each adjusted their currencies of pounds (£), shillings (s) and pence (d) to a decimalised format. Prior to that, a pound was made up of 20 shillings, each of which was made up of 12 pennies. The new, decimalised pound retained its value and name but was divided into 100 new pennies. Shillings disappeared. Similarly, a *tanner,* which was six old pennies, disappeared overnight.

10. Misplaced abbreviation: Mrs Margaret Murphy has told the story of her son's death due to mistakes in the transfer of critical information regarding a blood test for calcium levels. The image appears online and shows the actual notation, with abbreviations used. Mrs Murphy has since acted as a patient advocate and catalyst for improved standards relating to communicating patients' test results. https://improvement.nhs.uk/documents/1138/SLIDES_B2_W_Patient_exp_story_as_catalyst.pdf last accessed 1 Jan 2020, and at https://www.imt.ie/features-opinion/victim-of-a-killing-machine-05-05-2008/.

11. Medical eponyms. The following articles present differing opinions on this topic. Robertson, M. G. 'Fame is the spur the clear eponym doth raise'. *Journal of the American Medical Association*, 1972;221:1278; Rodin, A. E., Key, J. D. *Medicine, Literature and Eponyms: An Encyclopedia of Medical Eponyms Derived from Literary Characters.* Robert E. Krieger Publishing Company,

Malabar, Florida, 1989; Woywodt, A., Matteson, E. 'Should eponyms be abandoned? Yes.' *British Medical Journal,* 2007;335:424; Whitworth, J. A. 'Should eponyms be abandoned? No.' *British Medical Journal,* 2007;335:425; Jeffcoate, W. J. 'Should eponyms be actively detached from diseases?' *Lancet,* 2006; 367:1296-7; Woywodt, A., Lefrak, S., Matteson, E. 'Tainted eponyms in medicine: The "Clara" cell joins the list.' *European Respiratory Journal,* 2010;36:706-708;   Czech, H. 'Hans Asperger, National Socialism, and 'race hygiene' in Nazi-era Vienna.' *Molecular Autism,* 2018; 9:29; Sheffer, E. *Asperger's Children: The Origins of Autism in Nazi Vienna.* W. W. Norton & Company Ltd, London, 2018; Feinstein, Adam. *A History of Autism: Conversations with the Pioneers.* Wiley-Blackwell, Chichester, UK, 2010; Shanahan, F., Houlihan, C., Marks, J. C. In praise of the literary eponym – Henry V sign. *Quarterly Journal of Medicine,* 2013;106:93-94.

CHAPTER 3: THE ILLNESS WORDS

1. Dr Hacib Aoun died with AIDS following infection acquired accidentally from a broken glass vial of blood from an AIDS-infected patient.

2. Lee, T. H. 'The word that shall not be spoken'. *New England Journal of Medicine,* 2013;369:1777-79.

3. Groopman, Jerome. *The Anatomy of Hope: How People Prevail in the Face of Illness.* Random House Trade Paperbacks. New York, 2004.

4. 'An alternative view of suffering: Tate, Tyler and Pearlman, Robert. What we mean when we talk about suffering – and why Eric Cassell should not have the last word.' *Perspectives on Biological Medicine,* 2019;62:95-110.

5. Katherine Young analyses the doctor-patient interaction and describes a 'sense of loss of self' at the hands of dispassionate carers. 'Narrative Embodiments: Enclaves of the Self in the Realm of Medicine.' In *Texts of Identity,* ed. John Shotter and Kenneth J. Gergen. London: Sage, 1989, 153.

6. The case is cited by Ehrenreich and is based on an account by Jimmie Holland, a psychiatrist at Memorial Sloan Kettering Cancer Center, New York. Holland has written on 'The Tyranny of Positive Thinking' in *The Human Side of Cancer: Living with Hope, Coping with Uncertainty.* Holland, Jimmie C., and Lewis, Sheldon. Harper Collins, New York, 2000.

7. This topic was explored by interviewing patients with ulcerative colitis who were 'cured' by the creation of an ileostomy: Kelly, Michael. 'Self, identity and radical surgery'. *Sociology of Health and Illness,* 1992;14:390-415.

8. Concealment has featured in the accounts of illness for many politicians and celebrities. In some instances, the medical profession has been complicit, such as the secret surgery performed at sea on President Grover Cleveland, and the failure to comment on the adrenal glands and the possibility of

Addison's disease at the autopsy on President John Fitzgerald Kennedy. In the 1960s, the presence of illness would have been regarded as a weakness in a president and might have adversely affected JFK's prospects of re-election. Algeo, Mathew. *The President Is a Sick Man*, Chicago Review Press, Chicago: 2011; Bumgarner, John R. *The Health of the Presidents*. McFarland & Company, Inc. Jefferson, North Carolina and London, 1994; Gilbert, Robert E. *The Mortal Presidency: Illness and Anguish in the White House*. Fordham University Press, New York, 1998.

9.   The chronic illnesses of Charles Darwin are reviewed in Shanahan, Fergus, 'Darwinian dyspepsia: an extraordinary scientist, an ordinary illness, great dignity'. *American Journal of Gastroenterology*, 2012;107:161-4

10. Gain from illness is also discussed in O'Mahony, Seamus and Shanahan, Fergus, 'Ethereal and material gain: unanticipated opportunity with illness or disability'. *Clinical Medicine*, 2014;14:44-46.

11. Lee, Thomas H., McGlynn, Elizabeth A., Safran, Dana Gelb. 'A framework for increasing trust between patients and the organisations that care for them'. *Journal of the American Medical Association*, 2019;321: 539-540.

CHAPTER 4: WAITING, UNCERTAINTY AND TIME

1.   First published in *Hektoen International: A Journal of Medical Humanities*, Vol 5, Issue 3, Summer 2013

2.   Lawlor, Aine. In dialogue at *The Experience of Illness: Learning from the Arts, A symposium*, University College Cork, National University of Ireland, 30 Nov 2012.

3.   Christensen, J. The family in the waiting room. *Journal of General Internal Medicine*, 2007;22:1479

4.   Lara, F. *The Waiting Room*. http://www.short-story.net/read/1447/the-waiting-room2 (accessed 20 Feb 2013)

5.   Lowry, L. S.: The image of *A Doctor's Waiting Room* is depicted in Rohde, Shelley. *L. S. Lowry: A Biography*. Third edition. Salford: Lowry Press, 1999, and that of *Ancoats Hospital Outpatients Hall* appears in Sandling, Judith, Leber, Mike. *Lowry's City*. Salford: Lowry Press, 2000.

6.   Kirwan, Liam. *Political Correctness and the Surgeon*. Milton Keynes: AuthorHouse 2008, 33.

7.   Wellcome Collection, Ford, K. (curator) *Death: A Picture Album*. London: Wellcome Trust, 2012.

8.   Schweizer, H. *On Waiting: Thinking in Action*. London: Routledge, Taylor & Francis Group, 2008, 88.

9.   Uncertainty: the value of acknowledging uncertainty is further explored in the following articles. Han, P. K. J. 'The need for uncertainty: A case for

prognostic silence.' *Perspectives in Biological Medicine,* 2016;59:567-75; and Wellbery, C. 'The value of medical uncertainty?'. *Lancet* 2010;375: 1686-7.

10. 'The velocity of the ill, however, is like that of the snail.' Emily Dickinson in communication with Charles H. Clark, quoted in *Emily Dickinson and the Art of Belief* by Roger Lundin, Revised Edition 2004, Wm B Eerdmans Publishing Co., Grand Rapids, Michigan.

CHAPTER 5: IT'S THE WAY YOU SAY IT

1. William Carlos Williams. *Selected Essays.* New Directions Publishing Corporation, New York, 1969.

2. YouTube: What did you do to my sign? The Power of Words in Glasgow https://www.youtube.com/watch?v=pzjEzohHmaM. Last accessed 18 Jan 2020.

3. Only the names of the patients are fictitious; their words and stories are real.

4. My colleague Dr Gary Lee alerted me to the nuances of English as spoken in Cork. I had already been familiar with the Irish enrichment of the English language with Celtic words and expressions, much of which was explored in the famous television documentary and book *The Story of English* by Robert MacNeil, Robert McCrum and William Cran (New York: Viking, 1986). It has been claimed that if Shakespeare were alive today, he would be most at home in Cork, Ireland, because there he would find Elizabethan English preserved and blended with Gaelic.

5. The influence of language on voter turn-out at elections: Gilovich, Thomas, Ross, Lee. *The Wisest One in the Room.* Oneworld Publications, London, 2016; Bryan, C. J., Walton, G. M., Rogers, T., Dweck, C. S. 'Motivating voter turnout by invoking the self.' *Proceedings of the National Academy of Sciences, USA.* 2011;108(31):12653-6. doi: 10.1073/pnas.1103343108.

6. Sources on the influence of information framing: Gilovich, T., Ros,s L. *The Wisest One in the Room.* Oneworld Publications, London, 2016; Tversky A, Kahneman D. 'The framing of decisions and the psychology of choice'. *Science.* 1981, Jan 30;211(4481):453-8.;Tversky, A., Kahneman, D. 'Judgement under Uncertainty: Heuristics and Biases'. *Science.* 1974, Sep 27;185(4157):1124-31; Lewis, M. *The Undoing Project: A Friendship that Changed the World.* Allen Lane, Penguin Books, 2017, London.; McNeil, B. J., Pauker, S. G., Sox, H. C. Jr, Tversky, A. 'On the elicitation of preferences for alternative therapies.' *New England Journal of Medicine,* 1982 May 27;306(21):1259-62.; Perneger, T. V., Agoritsas, T. 'Doctors and patients' susceptibility to framing bias: a randomized trial'. *Journal of General Internal Medicine,* 2011;26:1411-17.

7. On interruptions in the patient-doctor interview: Mauksch, Larry B. 'Questioning a Taboo: Physicians' interruptions during interactions with

patients'. *Journal of the American Medical Association,* 2017;317:1021-1022; and associated correspondence: Physicians interrupting patients: *Journal of the American Medical Association,* 2017:318:92-95; Singh Ospina, N., Phillips, K. A., Rodriguez-Gutierrez, R., *et al.* 'Eliciting the Patient's Agenda: Secondary Analysis of Recorded Clinical Encounters'. *Journal of General Internal Medicine,* 2018: https://doi.org/10.1007/s11606-018-4540-5; and associated correspondence: Mohammed, R. S. D., Yeung, E. Y. H. 'Physicians interrupting patients'. *Journal of General Internal Medicine,* 2019 DOI: 10.1007/s11606-019-05140-1

8. Plain language is discussed in greater detail by Russell Willerton: *Plain Language and Ethical Action: A Dialogic Approach to Technical Content in the Twenty-first Century.* Routledge, Taylor & Francis Group, New York, 2015. Clean language is discussed in greater detail by Wendy Sullivan and Judy Rees: *Clean Language: Revealing Metaphors and Opening Minds.* Crown House Publishing Ltd, 2008, Camarthen, Wales. The concept of clean language was formulated by the late David Grove: 'And what kind of man is David Grove? An interview with Penny Tomkins and James Lawley.' https://www.cleanlanguage.co.uk/articles/articles/37/1/And-what-kind-of-a-man-is-David-Grove/Page1.html accessed 10 Dec 2019.

CHAPTER 6: NO WORDS, JUST SILENT SIGNALS

1. Christy Brown, an Irish poet and memoirist famous for his book *My Left Foot* and *Down All the Days,* wrote these words in the foreword to the autobiography by his paediatrician, Dr Robert Collis. Collis, Robert. 1975. *To Be a Pilgrim.* Secker & Warburg, London pIX.

2. The image appeared in an article by Dr Elizabeth Toll about the distancing effect of medical technology, particularly the electronic medical record: Toll, E. 'A piece of my mind: The cost of technology'. *Journal of the American Medical Association,* 2012;307:2497-8.

3. For further discussion of the importance of acting in doctoring: Finestone, H. M., Conter, D. B. 'Acting in medical practice'. *Lancet,* 1994;344:801-802; O'Donnell, Michael. 'Doctors as performance artists'. *Journal of the Royal Society of Medicine,* 2005;98:323-324; O'Donnell, Michael. 'The night Bernard Shaw taught us a lesson'. *British Medical Journal,* 2006;333:1338-1340; Sokol, Daniel K. 'Medicine as performance: What can magicians teach doctors?' *Journal of the Royal Society of Medicine,* 2008;101:443-446; Whorwell, P. J., Shanahan, F. 'In the performing art of medicine: the doctor as actor'. *Quarterly Journal of Medicine* 2015:1-2; Misch, Donald A. 'I feel witty, oh so witty'. *Journal of the American Medical Association,* 2016;315:345-6; Kneebone, Roger L. 'Performing magic, performing medicine'. *Lancet,* 2017; 389: 148-149.

Chapter 7: Healing Words, Hurtful Words

1. Shanahan F. First published 7 Jun 2016, in an open-access British Medcical Journal blog http://blogs.bmj.com/medical-humanities/2016/06/07/first-impressions-only-happen-once/1/

2. Cited by Daniel Corkery: *The Hidden Ireland: A Study of Gaelic Munster in the Eighteenth Century.* Gill and MacMillan, Dublin, 1967.

Chapter 8: Language Gaps and Words that Get in the Way

1. Wu, A. W. 'Medical error: the second victim. The doctor who makes the mistake needs help too'. *British Medical Journal,* 2000;320:726-7; Wu, A. W., Shapiro, J., Harrison, R., Scott, S. D., Connors, C., Kenney, L., Vanhaecht, K. 'The impact of adverse events on clinicians: What's in a name? *Journal of Patient Safety,* 2017 Nov 4. doi: 10.1097/PTS.0000000000000256; Grissinger, M. 'Too many abandon the "second victims" of medical errors'. *Pharmacy and Therapeutics,* 2014;39:591-2; Clarkson, M. D., Haskell, H., Hemelgarn, C., Skolnik, P. J. 'Abandon the term "second victim": an appeal from families and patients harmed by medical errors'. *British Medical Journal,* 2019;364:11233.

2. *Perpetual Disappointments Diary,* Nick Asbury. London: Boxtree Press, 2018.

Chapter 9: When Words Turn People into Patients

1. John Caffey, MD, is cited in the following historical perspective on the thymus gland: Jacobs, M. T., Frush, D. P., Donnelly, L. F. 'The right place at the wrong time: historical perspective of the relation of the thymus gland and pediatric radiology'. *Radiology,* 1999; 210:11-16.

2. 'What is Normal?' The difficulties defining *normal, health* and *disease* have been addressed by many authors but the following articles are particularly noteworthy: Davis, P. V., Bradley, J. G. 'The meaning of normal'. *Perspectives in Biological Medicine,* 1996;40:68-77; Fitzgerald, F. T. 'The tyranny of health'. *New England Journal of Medicine,* 1994;331:196-198; Davies, P. G. 'Between health and illness'. *Perspectives on Biological Medicine,* 2007;50:444-452; Dalrymple, T. 'Secular Salvation: Defining Health'. In Dalrymple, Theodore. *An Intelligent Person's Guide to Medicine.* Duckworth, London 2001; Smith, R. 'In search of "non-disease".' *British Medical Journal,* 2002; 324:883-885.

3. Skrabanek, P. 'Nonsensus consensus'. *Lancet,* 1990;335:1446-47.

4. Long after the publication of *Medical Nemesis,* Illich told one of his friends that the book was not specifically about medicine. His biographer, Todd Hartch, claimed that Illich's works, including *Medical Nemesis,* were really about the corruption of Christianity. This suggestion – that *Medical Nemesis* was more akin to a parable, or, as Illich himself would describe

it, 'apophatic' – doesn't ring true. The book was very specifically about medicine and was heavily annotated with detailed medical footnotes. Illich liked to throw people off the scent, and this is an example of his trickiness.

5.   World Health Organisation: 'Best practices for the Naming of New Human Infectious Diseases', May 2015. https://www.hst.org.za/publications/ NonHST%20Publications/WHO HSE FOS 15.1 eng.pdf last accessed 30 Dec 2019.

6.   The Lotronex story: (a) The original trial was published as follows: Camilleri, M., Northcutt, A.R., Kong, S., Dukes, G. E., McSorley, D., Mangel, A. W. 'Efficacy and safety of alosetron in women with irritable bowel syndrome: a randomised, placebo-controlled trial.' Lancet 2000;355:1035-40; (b) Subsequent commentary by the editor of *Lancet*: Horton, R. 'Lotronex and the FDA: a fatal erosion of integrity'. *Lancet,* 2001; 357:1544-45; (c) Adverse effects: Chang, L., Tong, K., Ameen, V. 'Ischaemic colitis and complications of constipation associated with the use of Alosetron under a risk management plan: clinical characteristics, outcomes, and incidences'. *American Journal of Gastroenterology,* 2010;105:866-875.

7.   Nickel, B., Barratt, A., Copp, T., Moynihan, R., McCaffery, K. 'Words do matter: a systematic review on how different terminology for the same condition influences management preferences'. *British Medical Journal, Open* 2017 Jul 10;7(7):e014129. doi: 10.1136/bmjopen-2016-014129.

CHAPTER 10: CARING, DIGNITY AND EMPATHY

1.   Ellman, Richard. *James Joyce.* New and revised edition. Oxford: Oxford University Press. 1982, 397.

2.   This piece was first published as: Shanahan, Fergus. 'The professor and the playwright on what it means to care'. *Hektoen International,* 2019; 11(3).

CHAPTER 11: LANGUAGE, LOGIC AND PUBLIC HEALTH POLICY

1.   Boswell, James. *Boswell's Life of Johnson.* Project Guttenberg https:// www.gutenberg.org/files/1564/1564-h/1564-h.htm accessed 21 Dec 2019

2.   Galea, Sandro. *Well: What We Need To Talk About When We Talk About Health.* Oxford: Oxford University Press, 2019.

3.   Finlay, B. Brett, Arrieta, Marie-Claire. *Let Them Eat Dirt: Saving Your child from an Oversanitized World.* Algonquin Books of Chapel Hill, Chapel Hill, USA, 2016; Gilbert Jack, Knight Rob with Blakeslee Sandra. *Dirt Is Good.* St Martin's Press, New York, 2017.

4.   On the dangers of the Hygiene Hypothesis: (a) Parker, W. 'The "hygiene hypothesis" for allergic disease is a misnomer'. *British Medical Journal,*

2014;349:g5267. doi: 10.1136/bmj.g5267; (b) Bloomfield, S. F., Rook, G. A. W., Scott, E. A., Shanahan, F., Stanwell-Smith, R., Turner, P. 'Time to abandon the hygiene hypothesis: new perspectives on allergic disease, the human microbiome, infectious disease prevention and the role of target hygiene'. *Perspectives in Public Health,* 2016;136:213-224.

5.   Obituary of Ellen Maud Bennett, published in *Victoria Times Colonist,* 14/15 Jul 2018. https://www.legacy.com/obituaries/timescolonist/obituary. aspx?n=ellen-maud-bennett&pid=189588876 accessed 21 Dec 2019.

6.   *Mail Online*: https://www.dailymail.co.uk/news/article-1298394/Call-overweight-people-fat-instead-obese-says-health-minister.html   accessed 22 Dec 2019.

7.   Puhl, R., Peterson, J. L., Luedicke, J. 'Motivating or stigmatizing? Public perceptions of weight-related language used by health providers'. *International Journal of Obesity* 2013;37:612-619.

8.   Mendelson, M., Balasegaram, M., Jinks, T., Pulcini, C., Sharland, M. 'Antibiotic resistance has a language problem'. *Nature,* 2017 May 3;545(7652):23-25.

9.   Horne, Z., Powell, D., Hummel, J. E., Holyoak, K. J. 'Countering antivaccination attitudes'. *Proceedings of the National Academy of Sciences, USA,* 2015, Aug 18;112(33):10321-4. PMID:26240325

CHAPTER 12: THE PATIENT AND THE SYSTEM

1.   *Medical-industrial complex*: this is somewhat analogous to the 'military-industrial complex' and refers to networks of providers of healthcare services and products for profit. The term was popularised by Dr Arnold Relman, a former editor of the *New England Journal of Medicine,* in an article in the same journal (1980;303:963-970), although the concept was first formulated by Barbara and John Ehrenreich.

2.   The influential annual Shattuck Lecture of the Massachusetts Medical Society, presented in 2019 by Dr John Noseworthy and published in the 5 December edition of the *New England Journal of Medicine* (2019;381:2265-69) is entitled 'The Future of Care: Preserving the Patient-Physician Relationship' and advocates for two principles that support the patient-physician relationship: that physicians be allowed adequate time with their patients, and that a coordinating physician be identified for all patients, particularly those with complex and multiple disorders that require effective communication among all of the carers involved.

3.   Francis, Robert. 'The Mid Staffordshire NHS Foundation Trust Public Inquiry'. 2013. https://assets.publishing.service.gov.uk/government/uploads/system/uploads/attachment_data/file/279124/0947.pdf   last accessed 18 Jan 2020.

4. Oxman, A. D., Sackett, D. L., Chalmers, I., Prescott, T. E. 'A surrealistic mega-analysis of redisorganisation theories'. *Journal of the Royal Society of Medicine,* 2006; 98:563-568.

5. Dictum usually attributed to Lucius Cary, 2nd Viscount Falkland (1610-43)

6. 'HSE Guidelines for Communicating Clearly using Plain English with our Patients and Service Users'. https://www.healthpromotion.ie/hp-files/docs/HNC01094.pdf accessed 16 Dec 2019.

7. George Orwell supposedly based his classic novel *1984* in large part on the bureaucratic language he encountered while working at the BBC. Discussed in 'Looking into the Abyss: George Orwell at the BBC', Fleay, C., Sanders, M. L., *Journal of Contemporary History,* Vol. 24, No. 3 (Jul 1989), 503-18.

8. Hill, A.P., Baeza, J. 'Dealing with things that go wrong'. *Lancet,* 1999;354:2099-10; Williams, B., Coyle, J., Healey, D. 'The meaning of patient satisfaction: an explanation of high reported levels'. *Society of Scientific Medicine,* 1998;47:1351-59.

Bibliography

Alda, Alan. *If I Understood You, Would I Have This Look on My Face? My Adventures in the Art and Science of Relating and Communicating.* New York: Random House, 2017. Print.

Angelou, Maya. http://www.oprah.com/omagazine/Oprah-Interviews-Maya-Angelou/1. http://davidkanigan.com/2013/03/03/peoplewill-never-forget-how-you-made-them-feel/. Last accessed 11 Feb 2015

Aoun, Hacib. 'From the eye of the storm, with the eyes of a physician.' *Annals of Internal Medicine,* 1992;16:335-38.

Armstrong, Lance. *It's Not About the Bike: My Journey Back to Life.* London: Yellow Jersey Press, 2001. Print.

Arnold, Mathew. *The Wish.* 1867 https://www.poemhunter.com/poem/a-wish/ last accessed 1 Jan 2019.

Asher, Richard. *Talking Sense.* London: Pitman Medical, 1972. Print.

Atwood, Margaret. *The Blind Assassin,* London: Virago Press, 2001. Print.

Auden, Wystan, H. *Collected Poems.* Ed. Edward Mendelson. New York: Random House USA, Inc., 2007. Print.

Bailey, Elizabeth Tova. *The Sound of a Wild Snail Eating.* Totnes, Devon: Green Books, 2010. Print.

Balint, Michael. *The Doctor, His Patient and the Illness.* Second edition. London: Pitman Medical, 1964. Print.

Beckett, Samuel. *Waiting for Godot.* Act 1. London: The Folio Society, 2000. Print.

Bennett, Alan. 'An average rock bun.' p599, *Untold stories.* Ed. Alan Bennett. London: Faber & Faber, 2005. Print.

——. *The Madness of George III.* London: Faber & Faber, 1995. Print.

——. *A Life Like Other People's*. London: Faber & Faber Ltd, 2009. Print.

——. *The Lady in the Van. The complete edition*. London: Faber & Faber Ltd, 2015. Print.

——. *Allellujah!* London: Faber & Faber Ltd, 2018. Print.

——. *Alan Bennett introduces Allelujah!* Bridge Theatre programme notes, London, 2018. Print.

Bennett, Amanda. *The Cost of Hope: The Story of Marriage, a Family, and the Quest for Life*. New York: Random House, 2012. Print.

Berger, John, Mohr, Jean. *A Fortunate Man*. New York: Holt, Rinehart & Winston, 1967. Print.

Biro, David. 'An Anatomy of Illness.' *Journal of Medical Humanities* 2012;33:41-54.

Bishop, Elizabeth. 'In the waiting room', *The Complete Poems*. New York: Farrar, Straus, and Giroux, 1983, 159.

Biss, Eula. 'The Pain Scale'. *Creative Nonfiction* No. 32, *The Best Creative Nonfiction Vol. 1* (2007), pp. 65-84. Print.

——. *On Immunity: An inoculation*. London: Fitzcarraldo Editions. 2015. Print.

——. 'Sentimental Medicine. Why we still fear vaccines.' *Harper's Magazine*, January 2013, 33-40. Print.

Blau, J. N. 'Clinican and Placebo.' *Lancet* 1985;325:344.

Bloom, Paul. *Against Empathy: The Case for Rational Compassion*. London: The Bodley Head, 2016. Print.

Blumhagen, Dan. 'Hyper-tension: A folk illness with a medical name.' *Culture, Medicine and Psychiatry* 1980;4:197-227.

Boswell, James. *Boswell's Life of Johnson*. Project Gutenberg https://www.gutenberg.org/files/1564/1564-h/1564-h.htm, accessed 21 Dec 2019.

Bound, Alberti F. *A Biography of Loneliness*. Oxford University Press. 2019.

Bourke, Joanna. *The Story of Pain: From Prayer to Painkillers*. Oxford: Oxford University Press, 2014. Print.

Bourke, Joanna. *Fear: A Cultural History*. London: Virago Press, 2005. Print.

Bowler, Kate. *Everything Happens for a Reason, and Other Lies I've Loved*. London: SPCK, 2018. Print.

Boyer, Anne. *The Undying: A Meditation on Modern Illness.* Allen Lane, London, 2019

Brennan, Frank. 'A short talk on hope.' *Illness, Crisis and Loss,* 2010;18:259-261.

——. 'The woman from county Meath.' *Annals of Internal Medicine,* 2006;144:11:864 also published In: *On Being a Doctor. 3.* Ed. Laine, C., LaCombe, M. A. Philadelphia: American College of Physicians, 2007. Print.

Brook, Robert H. 'A physician = emotion + passion + science'. *Journal of the American Medical Association,* 2010;304(22):2528-9. doi: 10.1001/jama.2010.1807. PMID: 21139114

Broyard, Anatole. *Intoxicated by My Illness, and Other Writings on Life and Death.* New York: Fawcett Columbine, 1992. Print.

Camus, Albert. *The Plague.* New York: Everyman's Library, 2004

Carel, Havi. *Illness: The Cry of the Flesh.* Third edition. London and New York: Routledge Taylor & Francis Group, 2019. Print.

Carlin, George. *George Carlin on soft language.* YouTube https://www. youtube.com/watch?v=o25I2fzFGoY, accessed August 26, 2019.

Caro, Robert A. 'Turn Every Page: A cub reporter, an old-timer's advice, and a lifetime of learning secrets.' The *New Yorker,* January 28, 2019. Print.

Carroll, Lewis. *The Annotated Alice: The definitive edition. Alice's Adventures in Wonderland and Through the Looking Glass.* Ed. Martin Gardner. London: Penguin Books, 2001. Print.

Cassell, Eric, J. 'The Nature of Suffering and the Goals of Medicine'. *New England Journal of Medicine,* 1982;306:639-45.

——. *The Nature of Suffering and the Goals of Medicine.* Second edition. Oxford: Oxford University Press, 2004. Print.

Charon, Rita. *Narrative Medicine: Honoring the Stories of Illness.* Oxford: Oxford University Press, 2006. Print.

Chaucer, Geoffrey, 'The Clerks Prologue', *The Riverside Chaucer,* Third edition. Ed. F.N. Robinson, Oxford: Oxford University Press, 2008. Print.

Colaianni, Allesandra. *The Language of Medicine.* p138-141. Ed. Laine, C., LaCombe, M. A. *On being a doctor,* vol 4. Philadelphia: American College of Physicians, 2014. Print.

Conan Doyle, Arthur. 'Silver Blaze'. *The Penguin Complete Sherlock Holmes*. London: Penguin, 2009. Print.

Conway, Kathlyn. *Beyond Words: Illness and the Limits of Expression*. Albuquerque: University of New Mexico Press, 2013. Print.

Collis, Robert. *To Be a Pilgrim*. London: Secker & Warburg, 1975. Print.

Couser, G. Thomas. *Signifying Bodies: Disability in Contemporary Life Writing*. Ann Arbor: University of Michigan Press, 2012. Print.

——. *Recovering Bodies: Illness, Disability and Life Writing*. Madison: University of Wisconsin Press, 1997. Print.

Cousins, Norman. 'Denial: Are Sharper Definitions Needed?' *Journal of the American Medical Association,* 1982;248:210-212.

——. *Anatomy of an Illness as Perceived by the Patient*. New York: Bantam Books, 1979. Print.

Czech, H. Hans Asperger, 'National Socialism, and "race hygiene" in Nazi-era Vienna'. *Molecular Autism,* 2018; 9:29

Dalrymple, Theodore. 'Of Horlicks and Heroism'. *New English Review*, May 2014 http://www.newenglishreview.org/Theodore_Dalrymple/Of_Horlicks_and_Heroism/ accessed 20 Feb 2018

——. *Life at the Bottom: The Worldview that makes the underclass*. Chicago: Ivan R. Dee Publishing, 2001. Print.

——. *An Intelligent Person's Guide to Medicine*. London: Duckworth, 2001. Print.

Darling, Julia, Fuller, Cynthia (eds). *The Poetry Cure*. Newcastle: Bloodaxe poetry series 3, 2005. Print.

Darling, Julia. 'A waiting room in August.' *The Poetry Cure*, Ed. Julia Darling and Cynthia Fuller. Newcastle: Bloodaxe poetry series 3, page 20, 2005. Print.

——. 'How to behave with the ill.' *The Poetry Cure*, Ed. Julia Darling and Cynthia Fuller. Newcastle: Bloodaxe poetry series, 3, 2005. Print.

——. 'Too Heavy.' *Indelible Miraculous: The collected poems of Julia Darling*. Ed. Bev Robinson. Todmorden, Lancashire: Arc Publications, 2015. Print.

Davidoff, F. 'Time' (Editorial). *Annals of Internal Medicine,* 1997;127:483-5.

de Beauvoir, Simone. *A Very Easy Death,* Trans. Patrick O'Brian, New York: Pantheon Books, 1964. Print.

DeForest, Anna. 'Better words for better deaths.' *New England Journal of Medicine,* 2019;380:211-13.

Diamond, John. '*C. Because Cowards Get Cancer Too . . .* ' London: Vermilion, 1998.

Dickens, Charles. *Little Dorrit,* Ware, Hertfordshire: Wordsworth Classics, 1996 (first published in 1857). Print.

Dickinson, Emily. *Selected Poems.* London: Folio Society, 2016. Print.

Donne, John. *Devotions Upon Emergent Occasions.* 1624. Available online at *Project Gutenberg* ebook https://www.gutenberg.org/files/23772/23772-h/23772-h.htm, XXIII. Meditation.

Doyle, Roddy. 'The Curfew.' The *New Yorker,* 2 Dec 2019. Print.

——. *The Guts.* London, UK: Jonathan Cape/Random House, 2013.

Dusenbery, Maya. *Doing Harm.* New York: Harper One, 2018, Print.

Dyer, E. L. 'Misunderstanding'. *Annals of Internal Medicine,* 1993; 118:647. Also published in *On Being a Doctor,* edited by Michael A. LeCombe, American College of Physicians, Philadelphia, 1995. Also available at http://collegeofphysicians.blogspot.com/2014/10/the-poetry-of-medicine.html Accessed 20 Aug 2019.

Edson, Margaret. *W;t.* London: Nick Hern Books, 1993. Print.

Ehrenreich, Barbara. 'Welcome to Cancerland: A mammogram leads to a cult of pink kitsch.' *Harper's Magazine.* Nov 2001;43-53.

——. *Smile or Die: How Positive Thinking Fooled America & the World.* London: Granta Publications, 2009. Print. This book was published in the USA under the title *Bright-Sided: How Positive Thinking is Undermining America.* New York: Picador, 2009. Print.

Eliot, Thomas Stearns. *Four Quartets.* http://www.paikassociates.com/pdf/fourquartets.pdf last accessed 16 Jan 2020.

Eliot, George. *The Mill on the Floss.* Ware: Wordsworth Classics. 1993. Print.

Ellman, Richard. *James Joyce.* New and Revised Edition. Oxford: Oxford University Press, 1982, 397. Print.

Fanthorpe, Ursula A. 'Waiting Room.' *The Poetry Cure.* Ed. Julia Darling and Cynthia Fuller. Newcastle: Bloodaxe poetry series:3, 19, 2005

——. 'For Saint Peter.' *U. A. Fanthorpe: New & Collected Poems.* Preface by Carol Ann Duffy. London: Enitharmon Press, 2010. Print.

Feinstein, Adam. *A History of Autism. Conversations with the Pioneers.* Chichester: Wiley-Blackwell, 2010. Print.

Fiedler, Leslie. 'The Tyranny of the Normal.' *The Hastings Center Report* (special supplement: 'On the care of Imperiled Newborns'), v. 14, n.2 (April 1984).

Fitzgerald, Faith T. 'A Tale of Two Patients.' *Annals of Internal Medicine*, 2004;140:929-930.

——. 'Curiosity.' *Annals of Internal Medicine*, 1999; 130:70-72.

Francis, Robert. 'The Mid Staffordshire NHS Foundation Trust Public Inquiry.' 2013. https://assets.publishing.service.gov.uk/government/uploads/system/uploads/attachment_data/file/279124/0947.pdf, last accessed 18 Jan 2020.

Frank, Arthur. *At the Will of the Body: Reflections on Illness.* Boston: Houghton Mifflin Company, 1991. Print.

Friel, Brian. *Translations.* London: Faber and Faber, 1981. Print.

Galasinski, Dariusz. 'Language Matters: A linguist's view on medicine.' *Sexually Transmitted Infections,* 2017;93:456-457.

Galea, Sandro. *Well: What We Need To Talk About When We Talk About Health.* Oxford: Oxford University Press, 2019. Print.

Gilligan, Vince, *Breaking Bad*, TV series, episode 1, series 1 (pilot) script, 2008: https://www.springfieldspringfield.co.uk/view_episode_scripts.php?tv-show=breaking-bad&episode=s01e01, accessed 9 Jan 2020.

Gilovich T, Ross L. *The Wisest One in the Room.* London: Oneworld Publications, 2016. Print.

Gladwell, Malcolm. *Blink: The Power of Thinking without Thinking.* New York: Little, Brown and Company, 2005. Print.

Gleeson, Sinéad. *Constellations: Reflections from life.* London: Picador, 2019. Print.

Goffman, Erving. *The Presentation of the Self in Everyday Life.* New York: Anchor Books, 1959. Print.

——. *Stigma: Notes on the Management of Spoiled Identity.* New York: Simon & Schuster Inc, 1963. Print.

Goldman, B. *The Secret Language of Doctors: Cracking the code of hospital culture.* Chicago: Triumph Books, 2014. Print.

Gould, Stephan Jay. 'The Median Isn't the Message. Virtual Mentor', *Americal Medical Association Journal of Ethics,* 2013;15(1):77-81. Reprinted from *Bully for Brontosaurus: Reflections in Natural History,* Stephen Jay Gould. Used with permission of the publisher, W. W. Norton & Company, Inc, 1991. Print.

Graham, Martha. 'Martha Graham Reflects on Her Art and a Life in Dance.' The *New York Times,* 31 March 1985. https://archive. nytimes.com/www.nytimes.com/library/arts/033185graham. html, accessed 9 Jan 2020.

Graziano, Michael S. A. *The Spaces Between Us: A Story of Neuroscience, Evolution and Human Nature.* Oxford: Oxford University Press, 2018. Print.

Grealy, Lucy. *Autobiography of a Face.* Boston: Mariner Books, 1994. Print.

Groopman, Jerome. *The Anatomy of Hope: How People Prevail in the Face of Illness.* New York: Random House Trade Paperbacks, 2004. Print.

Gunter, Jen. 'Medical misinformation and the internet: a call to arms.' *Lancet,* 2019;393:2294-2295

Hadler, Nortin. 'If you have to prove you are ill, you can't get well: the object lesson of fibromyalgia.' *Spine,* 1996;21:2397-2400.

Haines, Rainda (director). *The Doctor.* Touchstone Pictures Silver Screen Partners IV, 1991. Film.

Harrison, Jim. 'Larson's Holstein Bull'. In *In Search of Small Gods,* Port Townsend, WA: Copper Canyon Press, 2009

Hartch, Todd. *The Prophet of Cuernavaca: Ivan Illich and the Crisis of the West.* Oxford: Oxford University Press, 2015. Print.

Heaney, Seamus. 'Requiem for the Croppies.' *Seamus Heaney: 100 Poems.* London: Faber & Faber, 2018. Print.

——. in O'Driscoll, D. *Stepping Stones: Interviews with Seamus Heaney.* London: Faber and Faber, 2008. Print.

——. 'Miracle.' *The Human Chain.* London: Faber and Faber, 2010. Print.

Henderson, Lawrence J. 'Physician and patient as a social system.' *New England Journal of Medicine,* 1935;212:819-823.

Hill, Adam B. 'Breaking the stigma: a physician's perspective on self-care and recovery.' *New England Journal of Medicine,* 2017; 376:1103-1105.

Hitchens, Christopher. *Mortality*. London: Atlantic Books, 2012. Print.

Holland, Jimmie C. 'The Tyranny of Positive Thinking', *The Human Side of Cancer: Living with Hope, Coping with Uncertainty*. Eds. Jimmie C. Holland and Sheldon Lewis. New York: Harper Collins, 2000. Print.

Holmes Jr, O. W. 'Letter to Harold Laski, July 2nd 1917'cited in *The Oxford Dictionary of Humorous Quotations*. Ed. Sherrin N, Oxford: Oxford University Press, 1995, p166.

Hooper, Tom (director). *The King's Speech*. SeeSaw Films, UK Film Council, Bedlam Productions, 2010. Film.

Hopkins, Gerard Manley. 'Pied Beauty.' *Gerard Manley Hopkins: Poems and Prose*. London: Penguin Classics, 1985. Print.

Horton, Richard. 'Offline: Touch – the first language.' *Lancet*, 2019;394:1310

Hughes, Robert. *Things I Didn't Know*. New York: Vintage Books, A Division of Random House, Inc., 2006. Print.

Humphrys, John. *Lost for Words: The Mangling and Manipulating of the English language*. London: Hodder, 2005. Print.

——. *Beyond Words: How language reveals the way we live now*. London: Hodder & Stoughton, 2006. Print.

Humphrys, John, Jarvis, Sarah. *The Welcome Vistor: Living Well, Dying Well*. London: Hodder & Stoughton Ltd., 2009. Print.

Hunsaker Hawkins, Anne. *Reconstructing Illness: Studies in Pathography*. Second edition. West Lafayette, Indiana: Purdue University Press, 1999. Print.

Illich, Ivan. *Medical Nemesis: The Expropriation of Health*. London: Calder & Boyars Ltd, 1975. Print.

Jamison, Leslie. *The Empathy Exams: Essays*. London: Granta, 2014. Print.

Joyce, James. *Ulysses*. London: Penguin. 2000, 916. Print.

——. *Dubliners*. Ware: Wordsworth Classics, 1993. Print.

Judt, Tony. 'Night'. *Advances in Clinical Neuroscience and Rehabilitation*, 2010;10(1) March/April:22-23. Also published in the *New York Review of Books* (14 Jan 2010)

Kahneman, Daniel. *Thinking, Fast and Slow*. New York: Farrar, Straus and Giroux, 2011. Print.

Kavanagh, Patrick. *The Complete Poems*. Newbridge: The Goldsmith Press Ltd, 1972. Print.

Katz, Jay. *The Silent World of Doctor and Patient*. Baltimore: The Johns Hopkins University Press, 2002, p193-194. Print.

Kearney, M. *Mortality Wounded: Stories of Soul Pain, Death and Healing*. Dublin: Marino Books, 1996. Print.

Keller, Helen. *The World I Live In & Optimism: A Collection of Essays*. New York: Dover Publications Inc. Mineola, 2009. Print.

Khakpour, Porochista. *Sick: A Memoir*. Edinburgh: Canongate Books Ltd, 2018. Print.

Khullar, Dhruv. 'The Trouble with Medicine's Metaphors.' The *Atlantic*, 7 August 2014 https://www.theatlantic.com/health/archive/2014/08/the-trouble-with-medicines-metaphors/374982/, accessed 5 Dec 2019

——. Interviews. http://dhruvkhullar.com/interviews/, last accessed 13 Jan 2020.

Kleinman, Arthur. *The Illness Narratives: Suffering, Healing & the Human Condition*. New York: Basic Books, 1988. Print.

——. 'Catastrophe and caregiving: the failure of medicine as an art.' *Lancet* 371 (2008): 22-23.

——. 'Caregiving: the odyssey of becoming more human.' *Lancet* 373 (2009): 292-293.

——. 'Caregiving as moral experience.' *Lancet* 380 (2012): 1550-51.

——. 'How we endure.' *Lancet* 383 (2014): 119-120.

——. 'Care: in search of a health agenda.' *Lancet* 386 (2015): 240-241.

——. 'Presence.' *Lancet* 389 (2017): 2446-47.

——. 'The Soul in Medicine.' *Lancet* 394 (2019): 630-631.

Kneebone, Roger. 'Getting back in touch.' *Lancet* 391 (2018): 1348.

——. 'Performing magic, performing medicine.' *Lancet* 389 (2017): 148-149.

Kübler-Ross, Elizabeth. *On Death and Dying*. New York: Macmillan, 1969. Print.

Landau, Richard L. ' . . . And the Least of These is Empathy.' *Empathy and the Practice of Medicine*. Eds Howard Spiro, Mary McCrea Curnen, Enid Peschel, and Deborah St James. New Haven: Yale University Press, 1993. Print.

Larkin, Philip. 'Talking in Bed.' https://allpoetry.com/Talking-In-Bed accessed 30 Jan 2019

Launer, John. 'The three second consultation'. *Postgraduate Medical Journal,* 2009 Oct;85(1008):560. doi: 10.1136/pgmj.2009.088948.

Levine, Alexandra M. 'The Importance of Hope.' *Western Journal of Medicine,* 1989;150:609.

Lewis, M. *The Undoing Project: A Friendship that Changed the World.* London: Allen Lane, Penguin Books, 2017. Print.

Liao, Bill. 'On the importance of listening.' https://www.youtube.com/watch?v=ImHfNmA9F0s, last accessed on 9 Jan 2019

Lown, Bernard. *The Lost Art of Healing: Practising Compassion in Medicine.* New York: Ballantine Books, 1996. Print.

Luntz, Dr Frank. *Words that Work: It's Not What You Say, It's What People Hear.* New York: Hachette Books, 2007. Print.

Lynn, Jonathan and Jay, Antony. *The Complete Yes Minister.* London: BBC Books, 1989. Print.

MacIntyre, Alisdair. 'Seven traits for designing our descendants.' *Hastings Center Report* 9 (1979): 5-7.

Macklin, Ruth. 'Dignity is a useless concept.' *British Medical Journal,* 2003;327:1419-20.

Macnaughton, Jane. 'The dangerous practice of empathy.' *Lancet,* 2009;373:1940-41.

Mann, Thomas. *The Magic Mountain.* Trans. H. T. Lowe-Porter, London: Vintage, 1999. Print.

Manning, Kimberly D. 'The Nod.' *Journal of the American Medical Association,* 2014;312:133-134.

McCartney, Margaret. *The Patient Paradox.* London: Pinter & Martin Ltd, 2012. Print.

McCormick, James. 'The abuse of language and logic in epidemiology.' *Perspectives in Biological Medicine,* 1992;35(2)186-188.

McCrum, Robert. *My Year Off: Rediscovering Life after a Stroke.* London: Picador, 1998. Print.

McCullough, David. *Mornings on Horseback.* New York, Simon & Schuster Inc., 1981. Print.

McNeil, B. J., Pauker, S. G., Sox, H. C. Jr, Tversky, A. 'On the elicitation of preferences for alternative therapies.' *New England Journal of Medicine.* 1982 May 27;306(21):1259-62.

Medawar, Peter. 'Darwin's illness.' *The Strange Case of the Spotted Mice and Other Classic Essays on Science.* Oxford: Oxford University Press, 1996. Print.

Mendel, David. *Proper Doctoring.* New York: New York Review of Books, 2013. Print.

Middlebrook, Christina. *Seeing the Crab: A Memoir of Dying Before I Do.* New York: BasicBooks, 1996. Print.

Montagu, Ashley. *The Elephant Man: A study in human dignity.* New York: E. P. Dutton, 1979. Print.

Moore, Lorrie. 'People like that are the only people here: canonical babbling in Peed Onk.' In: *Lorrie Moore: The Collected Stories,* London: Faber and Faber, 2008. Print.

Mukherjee, Siddhartha. 'The One and the Many'. The *New Yorker*, 6 April 2020. Print.

Munthe, Axel. *The Story of San Michele.* London: John Murray, 1929. Print.

Murphy, Robert F. *The Body Silent: The different world of the disabled.* New York, London: W. W. Norton, 1990. Print.

Murray, Elspeth. *This is Bad Enough,* 2006, http://cancerconsortium.net/bad-enough-elspeth-murray/, accessed 11 Dec 2019.

O'Donnell, Michael. *Doctor! Doctor! An Insider's Guide to the Games Doctors Play.* London: Victor Gollancz Ltd, 1986. Print.

O'Driscoll, Denis. *Reality Check.* Port Townsend, Washington, Copper Canyon Press, 2008. Print.

Ofri, Danielle. *What Patients Say, What Doctors Hear.* Boston: Beacon Press, 2017, p174. Print.

O'Neill, Desmond. 'To live (and die) as an original.' *Journal of the American Medical Association,* 2012; 308:679-680.

Osler, William. *The Quotable Osler.* Eds. Mark E Silverman, T. Jock Murray, Charles S. Bryan. Philadelphia: American College of Physicians, 2008. Print.

Paling, John. 'Strategies to help patients understand risks.' *British Medical Journal,* 2003;327:745-748.

Papper, Solomon. 'Care of patients with incurable, chronic neoplasm: One patient's perspective.' *Americal Journal of Medicine,* 1985;78:271-276.

Payer, Lynn. *Disease-mongers: how doctors, drug companies, and insurers are making you feel sick.* New York: J. Wiley, 1992. Print.

Payne, Thomas. *Common Sense,* New York: Barnes and Noble Classics, 2005. Print.

Peabody, Francis W. 'The care of the patient.' *Journal of the American Medical Association,* 88 (1927): 877-882, and Rabin, P. L. and D. Rabin. 'The Care of the Patient. Francis Peabody Revisited.' *Journal of the American Medical Association* 252 (1984): 819-820.

Perkins, Gilman, Stetson, Charlotte, *The Yellow Wallpaper.* https://www.nlm.nih.gov/theliteratureofprescription/exhibitionAssets/digitalDocs/The-Yellow-Wall-Paper.pdf, accessed 28 Apr 2019.

Pine, Emilie. *Notes to Self.* Dublin: Tramp Press, 2018. Print.

Pinker, Steven. 'The stupidity of dignity.' The *New Republic,* 2008 https://newrepublic.com/article/64674/the-stupidity-dignity, accessed 29 Apr 2019.

Pope, Alexander. *An Essay on Man: Epistle I* https://www.poetryfoundation.org/poems/44899/an-essay-on-man-epistle-i, last accessed 12 Jan 2020.

Porter, Kathryn Anne. *Pale Horse, Pale Rider.* London: Penguin, 2011

Porter, Roy. *The Greatest Benefit to Mankind: A Medical History of Humanity.* New York, London: W. W. Norton & Company, 1997. Print.

Price, Reynolds. *A Whole New Life.* New York: Scribner, 1994. Print.

Pratchett, Terry. *Shaking Hands with Death.* London: Corgi Books, 2015. Print.

——. *A Slip of the Keyboard: Reflections on Life, Death and Hats.* London: Corgi Books, 2014. Print.

Proust, Marcel. *In Search of Lost Time: The Guermantes Way.* London: The Folio Society, 2005. Print.

Quigley, Columba. *The Good Death,* presented at a symposium entitled 'Ambiguities and Paradoxes in Clinical Practice', at the Centre for the Humanities and Health at King's College London, Salisbury Room, St Bride's Foundation, of Fleet Street, London, 27 September 2017.

Rabin, David, Rabin, Pauline L., Rabin, Roni. 'Compounding the ordeal of ALS: Isolation from my fellow physicians.' *New England Journal of Medicine,* 1982; 307:506-509.

Relman, Arnold. 'On Breaking One's Neck.' The *New York Review of Books*, 6 Feb 2014. Print.

Richards, Tessa. 'Chasms in communication still occur too often.' *British Medical Journal,* 1990;301:1407-1408.

Riess, Helen. *The Empathy Effect*. Boulder, Colorado: Sounds True, 2018. Print.

Robillard, Albert B. *Meaning of Disability: The Lived Experience of Paralysis*. Philadelphia: Temple University Press, 1999. Print.

Rodin, Alvin E, Key, Jack D. *Medicine, Literature and Eponyms: An Encyclopedia of Medical Eponyms Derived from Literary Characters*. Malabar, Florida: Robert E. Krieger Publishing Company, 1989. Print.

Rogers, Jenny, Maini, Arti. *Coaching for Health: Why It Works and How To Do It*. London: Open University Press, 2016. Print.

Rohde, Shelley. *L. S. Lowry: A biography*. Third edition. Salford: Lowry Press, 1999. Print.

Sacks, Oliver. *A Leg To Stand On*. London: Picador, 2012. Print.

Samuelson, Scott. *Seven Ways of Looking at Pointless Suffering*. Chicago and London: The University of Chicago Press, 2018. Print.

Sandling, Judith, Leber, Mike. *Lowry's City*. Salford: Lowry Press, 2000. Print.

Sapolsky, Robert M. 'Poverty's Remains.' *The Sciences*, September/October 1991:8-10.

——. *Why Zebras Don't Get Ulcers*. Third edition. New York: St. Martin's Griffin. 2004, p182-185. Print.

Schreiber, LeAnne. *Midstream: The Story of a Mother's Death and a Daughter's Renewal*. New York: Penguin Books, 1990. Print.

Schultz, Philip. *My Dyslexia*. New York: W. W. Norton & Company, 2011. Print.

Schwenk, T. L. 'Physician well-being and the regenerative power of caring.' *Journal of the American Medical Association*, 319 (2018):1543-44.

Selzer, Richard. 'Five Finger Exercises', *A Richard Selzer Reader: Blood and Ink*. Ed. Kevin Kerrane. Newark: University of Delaware Press, 2017. Print.

Shanahan, Fergus. 'Who needs doctors? Staying fresh in changing times.' *Clinical Medicine* 11 (2011): 587-588.

———. 'Darwinian dyspepsia: an extraordinary scientist, an ordinary illness, great dignity.' *American Journal of Gastroenterology,* 2012;107:161-4

———. 'The professor and the playwright on what it means to care.' *Hektoen International* 2019; 11(3).

Shaw, George Bernard. *Pygmalion.* London: Penguin Classics, 2000. Print.

Sheffer, E. *Asperger's Children: The Origins of Autism in Nazi Vienna.* London: W. W. Norton & Company Ltd, 2018. Print.

Shem, Samuel. *The House of God.* London: Black Swan, 1978. Print.

Shorter, Edward. *Bedside Manners: The Troubled History of Doctors and Patients.* New York: Simon and Schuster, 1985. Print.

Silverman, William A. 'The power of labels.' *Lancet,* 2004;364:929.

Simpson, R. R. *Shakespeare and Medicine.* Edinburgh and London, E. & S. Livingstone, Ltd, 1962. Print.

Skelton, John. 'Everything you were afraid to ask about communication skills.' *British Journal of General Practice,* 2005; 55:40-46.

———. *Language and Clinical Communication: This Bright Babylon.* Oxford: Radcliffe Publishing, 2008. Print.

Skrabanek, Petr, McCormick, James. *Follies & Fallacies in Medicine.* Glasgow: Tarragon Press; 1989. Print.

Skrabanek, Petr. 'False Premises False Promises', *Selected Writings of Petr Skrabanek,* introduction by George Davey Smith, Taragon Press for the Skrabanek Foundation https://euract.woncaeurope. org/sites/euractdev/files/documents/resources/documents/ falsepremisesfalsepromisespetrskrabanek-2000.pdf, accessed 21 Dec 2019.

Smith, Richard. 'In search of "non-disease".' *British Medical Journal,* 2002; 324:883-885.

———. 'It's hard, perhaps impossibly hard, to be a good doctor.' *British Medical Journal* blog, 11 June 2012. https://blogs.bmj.com/ bmj/2012/06/11/richard-smith-its-hard-perhaps-impossibly-hard-to-be-a-good-doctor/

Sokol, Daniel K. 'The death of DNR: Can a change of terminology improve end of life care?' *British Medical Journal*, 2009;338:1043.

Solnit, Rebecca. *Hope in Dark. Untold Histories, Wild Possibilities.* Third edition, Chicago, Illinois, Haymarket Books, 2016. Print.

Sontag, Susan. *Illness as Metaphor & AIDS and Its Metaphors.* London: Penguin Modern Classics, 1991. Print.

Specter, Michael. *Denialism: How Irrational Thinking Hinders Scientific Progress, Harms the Planet, and Threatens Our Lives.* New York: The Penguin Press, 2009. Print.

Spence, Jo, Dennett, Terry, Jacob, Clarissa, Tobin, Amy. *Jo Spence: The Final Project.* Ed. Lee Louisa, London: Ridinghouse, 2013. Print.

Spinney, Laura. *Pale Rider: The Spanish Flu of 1918 and How It Changed the World.* London: Vintage, 2017. Print

Spiro, H., McCrea, Curnen M., Peschel, E., and St James, D. (eds) *Empathy and the Practice of Medicine*, New Haven: Yale University Press, 1993. Print.

Street, Alice. 'Making people care.' *Lancet,* 387 (2016): 333-34.

Struth, Thomas. *The Dandelion Room.* New York: DAP/Distributed Art Publishers, 2001. Print.

Sullivan, John. *Only Fools and Horses.* Episode: 'Thicker than Water' (third Christmas special) Dir. Ray Butt. BBC, 1983. TV.

Sullivan, Wendy, Rees, Judy. *Clean Language: Revealing Metaphors and Opening Minds.* Camarthen, Wales: Crown House Publishing Ltd, 2008. Print.

Swift, Jonathan. 'In Sickness.' *The Poems of Jonathan Swift. Vol 1.* 1882: Press of C. Whittingham. Free Ebook. https://play. google.com/store/books/details?id=SyhAAAAAYAAJ&rdid=book-SyhAAAAAYAAJ&rdot=1, last accessed 13 Jan 2020.

Taleb, Nassim Nicholas. *The Black Swan: The impact of the highly improbable.* New York: Random House, 2007. Print

——. *Skin in the Game: Hidden Asymmetries in Daily Life.* London: Allen Lane Penguin Books, 2018. Print.

Tanner, Laura E. 'Bodies in waiting: representations of medical waiting rooms in contemporary American fiction.' *American Literary History,* 2002;14(1):115-130.

Tavris, Carol. *Anger: The Misunderstood Emotion.* Revised Edition. New York: Touchstone, Simon & Schuster Inc., 1989. Print.

Thomas, Dylan. 'Do not go gentle into that good night.' https://allpoetry.com/do-not-go-gentle-into-that-good-night, accessed 13 Jan 2020

Thomas, Lewis. *The Medusa and the Snail: More Notes of a Biology Watcher.* New York: Viking Press, 1979. Print.

——. *The Youngest Science: Notes of a Medicine-Watcher.* Toronto: Bantham Books, 1983. Print.

Tolstoy, Leo. 'The Death of Ivan Ilyich.' Trans. Hugh Aplin. London: One World Classics Ltd. 2011, first published in Russian in 1886. Print.

Trollope, Anthony. *Doctor Thorne.* Ware: Wordsworth Classics. 2016, p108. Print.

Tversky Amos, Kahneman Daniel. 'Judgment under Uncertainty: Heuristics and Biases.' *Science,* 1974;185(4157):1124-31.

——. 'The framing of decisions and the psychology of choice.' *Science,* 1981 Jan 30;211(4481):453-8.

Twitchell, James B. *Twenty Ads That Shook the World: The Century's Most Groundbreaking Advertising and How It Changed Us All.* New York: Crown, 2000, pp60-69. Print.

Unger, Jim. *Herman: The Fourth Treasury.* Kansas City: Andrews and McMeel, Inc., 1984. Print.

Updike, John. 'At War with My Skin.' *Self-Consciousness: Memoirs by John Updike.* New York: Alfred A. Knopf, 2006. Print.

——. *From the Journal of a Leper.* Ed. C. Carduff. *John Updike Collected Later Stories,* New York: The Library of America, 2013. Print.

Watts, David. 'Silence knows the right questions', *The Orange Wire Problem and Other Tales from the Doctor's Office.* p53-66. Iowa City: University of Iowa Press, 2009. Print.

Watts, George Frederic. *Hope.* 1986 In: Nigel Llewellyn and Christine Riding (eds.), *The Art of the Sublime,* Tate Research Publication, January 2013, https://www.tate.org.uk/art/research-publications/the-sublime/george-frederic-watts-hope-r1105604, accessed 07 June 2020.

Weed, Larry L. *Medical Records, Medical Education and Patient Care.* Chicago: The Press of Case Western Reserve University, 1969. Print.

——. *Medicine in Denial.* Scotts Valley, California: Createspace, 2013. Web.

Weinberg, Richard B. 'The laying on of hands.' Ed. Michael A. LaCombe. *On Being a Doctor.* Philadelphia: American College of Physicians, 1995. Print.

——. 'Communion.' *On Being a Doctor 2.* Ed. Michael A. LaCombe, Philadelphia: American College of Physicians, 2000. Print.

Weinstein, Edwin A. *Woodrow Wilson: A Medical and Psychological Biography. Supplementary Volume to the Papers of Woodrow Wilson.* Princeton, New Jersey: Princeton University Press, 1981. Print.

Wilde, Oscar. *The Picture of Dorian Gray.* London: Folio Society, 2009. Print.

Willerton, Russell. *Plain Language and Ethical Action: A Dialogic Approach to Technical Content in the Twenty-First Century.* New York: Routledge, Taylor & Francis Group, 2015. Print.

Williams, William Carlos. *Selected Essays.* New York: New Directions Publishing Corporation, 1969.

——. *William Carlos Williams: The Doctor Stories,* Ed. Robert Coles, New York: New Directions Books, 1984. Print.

Wolfe, Thomas. *Look Homeward, Angel.* http://gutenberg.net.au/ebooks03/0300721.txt.

Woolf, Virginia. *On Being Ill.* Ashfield, Mass: Paris Press, 2012. Print. (first published in 1930).

Yeats, William B. *Selected Poems.* London: Folio Society, 1998. Print.

——. 'Easter 1916' http://www.theatlantic.com/past/docs/unbound/poetry/soundings/easter.htm, accessed 25 Feb 2013.

Acknowledgements

The idea for this book came in waves throughout my career, and was influenced by the patients with whose care I was privileged to be entrusted. I also benefited enormously while working with wonderful physicians and trainees. To all of my colleagues, now and in the past, I am grateful.

Without the encouragement and guidance of Seán O'Keeffe at Liberties Press this book might still be in a computer file marked 'unfinished projects'. Special gratitude goes to Marion Hassett, who patiently drew several images based on vague descriptions from me when words failed. I am deeply grateful to Elspeth Murray, who kindly granted permission to reproduce her poem 'This Is Bad Enough' in its entirety. I am also grateful to the following artists for granting permission to use images of their wonderful works: James and Michael Fitzgerald (The Project Twins), Tamsin van Essen, Nicholas Nixon, Paul Seawright and the Ryerson Image Center on behalf of the late Jo Spence. Dr Columba Quigley selflessly shared her thoughts on the illness-words, palliative medicine and much more on the experience of illness.

Prof. David Rampton in London was hugely encouraging at a time when I was unsure; he offered several helpful suggestions and corrected errors in the first draft. Prof. Patangi K. Rangachari at McMaster University, Canada, also offered numerous helpful suggestions. Special credit must go to Drs Eamonn Quigley in Houston and Peter Anton at UCLA, both of whom spent many hours talking and living medicine with me.

The following clinicians offered helpful suggestions and encouragement: John Sotos, Gary Lee, Charles Marks, Liam Farrell, Paula O'Leary and Dermot Ryan. A special word of thanks goes to my great friend and colleague Prof. Michael G. Molloy. For administrative and secretarial support, and much patience, I thank Rita Lynch and

Rosarie Daly. I also thank my friends and colleagues at APC Microbiome Ireland for their support over the past two decades. A special thanks also to Prof. Fiona Kearney and Chris Clarke at the Glucksman Gallery, University College Cork, Ireland. Last, but never least, I thank my wife Nora and my daughter Rosie for their support, constructive critiques, and practical help.

Index

AIDS 107, 189, 211

Alberti, Fay Bound 46, 198

Alda, Alan 153, 197

Alice in Wonderland 62, 69, 143, 165, 199,

Alzheimer's disease 38, 52, 147

Andersen, Hans Christian 32

Angelou, Maya 104, 197

anti-microbial resistance 160,

anxiety 5, 30, 34, 39, 103, 131, 138, 142, 143, 156

Aoun, Hacib 28, 32, 189, 197

Armstrong, Lance 49, 197

Arnold, Mathew 11, 197

Asher, Richard 13, 23, 129, 132, 197

Asperger's syndrome 21, 22, 189, 210

asthma 49, 130

Atwood, Margaret 99, 197

Auden, W. H. 44, 61, 197

autism 21, 162, 189, 200, 202, 210

bacteria 12, 47, 116, 160, 161, 184

Balint, Michael 35, 197

Bandaged heart (artwork) 109

Beckett, Samuel 54, 58, 197

Bennett, Alan 34, 99, 111, 146-8, 154, 197-8

Bennett, Amanda 29, 198

Berger, John (*A Fortunate Man*) 59, 62, 198

Betjeman, John 29, 45

Biro, David 44, 198

Bishop, Elizabeth 55, 198

Biss, Eula 122-3, 152, 163, 198

Blau, J. N. 105, 198

Bloom, Paul 152-3, 198

Blumhagen, Dan 121, 198

Bourke, Joanna 34, 122, 198

Bowler, Kate 7, 126, 199

Boyer, Anne 26, 36, 123, 165, 199

Breaking Bad (TV show) 89, 202

breast cancer 6, 11, 26, 27, 36, 54, 81, 107, 110, 126, 130, 165

Brennan, Cecily 109

Brennan, Frank 30, 199

Brook, Robert 2, 199

Brown, Christy 83, 216

Broyard, Anatole 2, 7, 54, 84, 95, 96, 108, 199

burnout 95, 99, 148, 165

Burroughs, William S. 138

Caffey, John 130, 193

Cameron, Norman 139

Camus, Albert 24, 178, 183, 185, 199

Canterbury Tales 77, 200
Carel, Havi 6, 32, 48, 150, 199
Carlin, George 124, 199
Caro, Robert A. 92, 199
Carroll, Lewis 119, 145, 199
Cassell, Eric 31, 32, 189, 199
Charon, Rita 93, 200
Chaucer 77, 200
Churchill, Winston 106
Clostridium difficile 161
Colaianni Allessandra 12, 199
Conan Doyle, Arthur 92, 199
Conway, Kathlyn 4, 40, 199
coping 1, 11, 17, 19, 39, 46, 59, 106, 108, 110, 145, 146, 147, 149, 150, 189, 204
Couser, Thomas 4, 43, 200
Cousins, Norman 38, 46, 50, 200
Covid-19 96, 158, 176-185
CPE (carbipenim-resistant enterococci) 116, 161
Crohn, Burrill 21
Crohn's disease 14, 21, 65, 66, 69
Crystal, David 15
Czech, Herwig 22, 189, 200

Dalrymple, Theodore 82, 113, 139, 173, 193, 200
Dalziel, T. K. 21
Darling, Julia 6, 11, 55, 200, 201
Darwin, Charles 17, 18, 47, 49, 190, 207, 210
Davidoff, Frank 60, 200
de Beauvoir, Simone 41, 201
DeForest, Anna 128, 201
delirium 18
dementia 35, 37
depression 35, 38, 39, 106, 115, 146, 179

diabetes 159
Diamond, John 111, 201
Dickens, Charles 22, 61, 173, 174, 201
Dickinson, Emily 27, 48, 61, 63, 116, 123, 124, 128, 191, 201
DNR ('Do Not Resuscitate') 127, 211
Doctor, The (film) 54, 202
Donne, John 5, 45, 62, 83, 201
Donnelly, William J. 17, 187, 188
Dorian Gray syndrome 22, 101, 213
Downton Abbey (TV show) 179
Doyle, Roddy 52, 107, 201
Drucker, Peter 92
Dusenbery, Maya 48, 201
Dyer, Eric 20, 201

Edson, Margaret 11, 26, 42, 107, 150, 201
Ehrenreich, Barbara 36, 49, 126, 135, 189, 195, 201
Eliot, George 106, 201
Eliot, T. S. 124, 201

Fanthorpe, Ursula A. 55, 201
Fauci, Anthony 182
Feinstein, Adam 22, 189, 202
fibromyalgia 136, 203
Fiedler, Leslie 131, 202
Fitzgerald, Faith 174, 193, 202
Flaubert, Gustave 24
Fracastoro, Girolamo 23
Francis report 168, 195, 202
Frank, Arthur 4, 48, 202
Friel, Brian 7, 119, 202

Galasinski, Dariusz 70, 202
Gardot, Melody 50

Gilman, Charlotte Perkins 119, 208
Gladwell, Malcolm 88, 202
Gleeson, Sinéad 12, 32, 42, 47, 123, 202
Goffman, Erving 86, 95, 112, 203
Goldacre, Ben 135
Gore, Al 77
Gould, Stephen Jay 117, 203
Goya, Francisco 24
Graham, Martha 85, 203
Graziano, Michael 98, 203
Grealy, Lucy 8, 43, 44, 50, 98, 203
Gunter, Jen 81, 82, 203

Harrison, Jim 178, 203
Havisham, Miss 61
Heaney, Seamus 7, 8, 28, 203
Heath, Iona 135
Helicobacter pylori 131, 156
Henderson, Lawrence J. 101, 116, 204
Henry V sign 24, 189
hepatitis 66, 67, 178
herd immunity 163, 177, 183
Higgins, Michael D. 178
Hill, Adam 115, 196, 204
Hitchens, Christopher 7, 8, 32, 46, 110, 112, 204
Hodler, Ferdinand 58
Hopkins, Gerard Manley 111, 112, 204
Horton, Richard 99, 194, 204
Hughes, Robert 46, 204
Humphrys, John 15, 58, 168, 204
Humpty Dumpty 69, 119, 165
Hunsaker Hawkins, Anne 4, 40, 204

hygiene hypothesis 157, 158, 194

I, Daniel Blake (film). 174, 202
Illich, Ivan 134-5, 193, 194, 203
infertility 127
inflammatory bowel disease 14, 65, 66
influenza 178-81,
Ionesco, Eugene 78
irritable bowel syndrome 18, 73, 136, 140-2, 194

Jamison, Leslie 154, 204
Jay, Antony 170, 187
Johnson, Samuel 154, 194, 198
Joyce, James 10, 52, 91, 92, 105, 129, 145, 194, 201
Judt, Tony 32, 34, 62, 204

Kahneman, Daniel 71, 102, 191, 205, 212
Katz, Jay 78, 205
Kavanagh, Patrick 106, 205
Kearney, Michael 32, 205,
Keller, Helen 97, 205
Khakpour, Porochista 47, 48, 205
Khullar, Dhruv 51, 108, 205
Kleinman, Arthur 2, 5, 8, 40, 99, 146, 147, 148, 205
Kneebone, Roger 87, 97, 192, 205
Kübler-Ross, Elizabeth 38, 205

Landau, Richard L. 154, 205
Larkin, Philip 37, 117, 206
Launer, John 87, 206
Le Carré, John 93
Lee, Gary 68, 191
Leśniowski, Antoni 21
Levine, Alexandra 29, 206
Liao, Bill 92, 206

Lister, Joseph 139
Loach, Ken 173, 174, 202
Loeffler, Imre 135
Lotronex (alesetron) 140-2, 194
Lown, Bernard 20, 96, 97, 101, 122, 135, 138, 206
Lowry, L. S. 56, 190, 209
Luntz, Frank 166, 206
Lyme disease 47
Lynn, Jonathan 170, 206

MacIntyre, Alisdair 27, 206
Macklin, Ruth 149, 150, 206
Macnaughton, Jane 151-2, 206
Madonna 184
Maini, Arti 76, 209
Mann, Thomas 62, 206
Manning, Kimberly 83, 84, 206
Marks, Charles 23, 24, 189
Maverick, Maury 170
McCartney, Margaret 93, 187, 206
McCormick, James 157, 206, 210
McCrum, Robert 33, 46, 54, 112, 191, 206
McCullough, David 49, 206
McLuhan, Marshall 117
Meadow, Roy 23
Medawar, Peter 47, 176, 207
medical-industrial complex 135, 165, 195
Mendel, David 5, 90, 207
mesothelioma 117
microbe, microbes 157, 158, 160, 161, 176, 182, 184, 185
Middlebrook, Christina 126, 207
Milton, John 38
Montagu, Ashley 150, 207
Moore, Lorrie 11, 37, 44, 71, 87, 110, 207

motor neurone disease 32, 38, 62, 114
Moynihan, Ray 135, 207
Mr D. 84
MRSA 116
Mukherjee, Siddhartha 182, 274
Munch, Edvard 179
Munchausen syndrome 23
Munthe, Axel (*The Story of San Michele*). 131, 132, 207
Murphy, Robert (*The Body Silent*) 44, 207
Murray, Elspeth 79, 207, 214

Nightingale, Florence 119
Nixon, Nicholas 97, 214

Obama, Barak 13, 166
obesity 8, 22, 159, 160, 161, 195
oesophageal cancer 7, 110
O'Donnell, Michael 94, 132, 192, 207
O'Driscoll, Denis 109, 203, 207
Ofri, Danielle 97, 98, 207
Ogburn, Charlton 167
O'Neill, Des 18, 207
Only Fools and Horses 120, 211
Orwell, George viii, 167, 196
Osler, William 28, 58, 133, 137, 150, 207
O'Toole, Fintan 50
ovarian cancer 11, 150

pain 14, 17, 30, 31, 32, 35, 43, 47, 61, 62, 66, 70, 99, 103, 105, 122, 123, 124, 138, 141, 151, 152, 179, 198, 205
Paling, John 72, 207
Papper, Solomon 151, 208
Paradise Lost 38

paralysis 33, 39, 209
Patchett, Ann 44
Payer, Lynn 135, 208
Payne, Thomas 13, 208
Peabody, Francis 148, 150, 208,
peptic ulcer 156
Petronius, Gaius 167
Pickwickian syndrome 22
Pine, Emilie 127, 208
Pinker, Steven 149, 208
Pollyanna syndrome 22
polycystic ovary syndrome 142,
    143
Pope, Alexander 27, 208
Porter, Eleanor H. 22
Porter, Katherine Anne 179, 208
Porter, Roy 5, 133, 208
psoriasis 42
Pratchett, Terry 38, 208
Price, Reynolds 33, 35, 208
Primum non nocere 10, 116, 187
Project Twins vii, 214
prostate cancer 2, 7
Proust, Marcel 24, 95, 119, 208
PTSD (post-traumatic stress
    disorder) 124
Pygmalion 113, 187, 210

Quigley, Columba 127, 128, 208

Rabin, David Dr 114, 209
Rather, Dan 143
Reiter's syndrome 21
Relman, Arnold 62, 135, 195, 209
Richards, Tessa 113, 187, 209
Robillard, Albert B. 38, 209
Rogers, Jenny 76, 209
Roosevelt, Theodore 49

Sacks, Oliver 33, 41, 42, 209

Samuelson, Scott 31, 209
Sapolsky, Robert A. 130, 209
Schreiber, Le Ann 41, 209
Schultz, Philip 49, 50, 209
science vii, viii, 2, 14, 26, 37, 58,
    78, 101, 116, 135, 137, 139,
    144, 153, 162, 166, 167, 181,
    182, 186, 191, 195, 197, 199,
    207, 209, 212
Seawright, Paul 56, 57
Shakespeare, William 24, 85, 95,
    132, 191, 210
Shaw, George Bernard 113, 187,
    192, 210
Sheffer, Edith 22, 189, 210
Shem, Samuel (*The House of God*)
    19, 188, 210
Shorter, Edward 175, 210
Silverman, William A. 130, 210
Simenon, Georges 92
Skelton, John 94, 210
Skrabanek, Petr 133, 135, 157,
    193, 210
Smith, Richard 2, 135, 136, 193,
    211
Sokol, Daniel 127, 192, 211
Solnit, Rebecca 28, 211
Sontag, Susan 107, 108, 211
soul 2, 32, 99, 205
Specter, Michael 162, 211
Spence, Jo 27, 36, 37, 211
Spinney, Laura 211
status thymolymphaticus 130
Strachan, David 158
stress 19, 35, 47, 71, 76, 89, 103,
    106, 121, 122, 124, 130, 139,
    144
stroke 7, 8, 31, 33, 39, 46, 112,
    206
Struth, Thomas 58, 110, 211

Swift, Jonathan 45, 211

Taleb, Nassim, Nicholas 89, 90, 181, 211
Tanner, Laura 54, 212
Tavris, Carol 35, 212
The Elephant Man (film) 159, 207
The King's Speech (film) 52, 112, 202
Thomas, Dylan 37, 212
Thomas, Lewis 97, 137, 212
Tolstoy, Leo 24, 33, 40, 45, 51, 212
Tova Bailey, Elizabeth 61, 197
Trollope, Anthony 98, 212
Trump, Donald 166
Tversky, Amos 71, 72, 102, 191, 207, 212
Twitchell, James B. 139, 212

ulcerative colitis 14, 189
Unger, Jim (*Herman* series) 22, 212
Updike, John 42, 212

vaccine, vaccination 8, 154, 161-3, 177, 195, 198
van Essen, Tamsin 180, 214
Victoria, Queen 61, 98, 119, 131, 195
Voltaire 60

Watts, David 94, 212
Watts, G. F. 28, 213
Wegener's granulomatosis 21
Weinberg, Richard 66, 97, 213
Weinstein, Edwin 39, 213
Wendell Holmes, Oliver 16
West, Mae 85
Wilde, Oscar 22, 101, 213

Williams, William Carlos 64, 122, 191, 213
Wilms' tumour 11
Wilson, Woodrow 39, 213
Wing, Lorna 21
Wolfe, Thomas 178, 213
Woolf, Virginia 119, 213
World Health Organisation (WHO) 143, 176, 177, 194

Yeats, W. B. 58, 105, 213
Yes Minister (TV show) 170, 206

zoonosis 177